100 CASES
in Dermatology

100 CASES
in Dermatology

Rachael Morris-Jones PhD PCME FRCP
Consultant Dermatologist & Honorary Senior Lecturer, King's College
Hospital, London, UK

Ann-Marie Powell
Consultant Dermatologist, St John's Institute of Dermatology, Guy's and St Thomas'
NHS Trust, London, UK

Emma Benton MB ChB MRCP
Post-CCT Clinical Research Fellow, St John's Institute of Dermatology,
Guy's and St Thomas' NHS Trust, London, UK

100 Cases Series Editor:
Professor P John Rees MD FRCP
Dean of Medical Undergraduate Education, King's College London School
of Medicine at Guy's, King's and St Thomas' Hospitals, London, UK

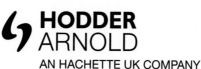

HODDER
ARNOLD
AN HACHETTE UK COMPANY

First published in Great Britain in 2011 by
Hodder Arnold, an imprint of Hodder Education, a division of Hachette UK
338 Euston Road, London NW1 3BH

http://www.hodderarnold.com

Hachette UK's policy is to use papers that are natural, renewable and recyclable products and made from wood grown in sustainable forests. The logging and manufacturing processes are expected to conform to the environmental regulations of the country of origin.

Whilst the advice and information in this book are believed to be true and accurate at the date of going to press, neither the author[s] nor the publisher can accept any legal responsibility or liability for any errors or omissions that may be made. In particular, (but without limiting the generality of the preceding disclaimer) every effort has been made to check drug dosages; however it is still possible that errors have been missed. Furthermore, dosage schedules are constantly being revised and new side-effects recognized. For these reasons the reader is strongly urged to consult the drug companies' printed instructions, and their websites, before administering any of the drugs recommended in this book.

British Library Cataloguing in Publication Data
A catalogue record for this book is available from the British Library

Library of Congress Cataloging-in-Publication Data
A catalog record for this book is available from the Library of Congress

ISBN-13   978-1-444-11793-6

1 2 3 4 5 6 7 8 9 10

Commissioning Editor: Joanna Koster
Project Editor: Stephen Clausard
Production Controller: Jonathan Williams
Cover Design: Amina Dudhia
Indexer: Laurence Errington

Typeset in 10/12 Rotis Serif by MPS Limited, a Macmillan Company, Chennai, India
Printed and bound in India

What do you think about this book? Or any other Hodder Arnold title?
Please visit our website at www.hoddereducation.com

CONTENTS

Contents

PREFACE

Dermatology is a broad and hugely enthralling specialty, where a clinician can actually visualize disease patterns up close – 'in the flesh'. In many ways dermatology is the art of the 'old-fashioned physician' who relies on careful history-taking and a thorough examination to make the majority of diagnoses. For the non-specialist, dermatological 'spot' diagnoses made through pattern-recognition alone can be challenging; therefore, this book strives to offer 'classic' presentations of common skin disorders through the fundamental tools of medicine – namely, a detailed history and observed clinical signs.

Part of the fascination with dermatological disorders is the ability of a physician to diagnose systemic disease through the observation of changes in the skin. Consequently, the accurate recognition of skin disorders is pertinent to all physicians in whatever field of medicine/surgery they are practising. Therefore, the cases selected in this book mainly reflect the interface between internal medicine and dermatology. It is often said that a picture is worth a thousand words; therefore, we hope that the clinical photographs accompanying each case will speak for themselves in many more words than we would ever be permitted to write.

Rachael Morris-Jones
Ann-Marie Powell
Emma Benton

ACKNOWLEDGEMENTS

The authors are indebted to all the patients who kindly allowed us to include their pictures in this book to illustrate the clinical signs. We would also like to sincerely thank the Medical Photography Departments in the St John's Institute of Dermatology, Guy's and St Thomas' Hospital NHS Trust and King's College Hospital NHS Trust for taking such excellent quality clinical images; and for the crucial role this plays in patient care and supporting ongoing Medical Education.

GLOSSARY

Abscess: deep collection of pus caused by a skin infection

Angioedema: temporary, rapid swelling of the skin

Annular: ring-shaped lesion

Atrophy: loss of tissue density

Bulla (-ae): large, fluid-filled blister(s) greater than 0.5 cm

Crust: dried skin fluid

Cyst: distinctive, closed sac-like structure in the skin, usually fluid with a semi-solid substance

Dermographism: 'writing on the skin', red, raised and inflamed skin due to firm stroking

Desquamation: peeling of superficial scales

Ecchymoses: bruise; a collection of blood in the skin

Emollient: moisturizer to soften and soothe the skin

Eroded: superficial loss of the epidermis

Excoriations: scratch marks causing partial/complete loss of the epidermis

Fissures: slits through the whole thickness of the skin

Fitzpatrick skin type: numerical classification of skin colour from type I (white) to type VI (black)

Fomites: inanimate object able to carry and hence transfer infectious particles

Furuncles: deep boil (skin infection) affecting the entire hair follicle

HAART: highly active antiretroviral therapy

Hyperkeratosis: thickening of the epidermis (stratum corneum)

Hypertrichosis: hair growth perceived to be excessive on the skin

Induration: hardening of the skin (e.g. due to inflammation, accumulation of fluid or tumour cells)

Koebner's phenomenon: skin lesions appearing in the lines of trauma

Lentigines: small area of increased pigmentation of the skin

Lichenification: thickening of the skin with prominent skin markings

Maceration: continually wet skin turns soft and white

Macule: change in the pigmentation of the skin (colour change) without any elevation (non-palpable)

Nikolsky's sign: sloughing-off of the epidermis from the dermis caused by lateral pressure

Nodule: circumscribed raised lesion greater than 1.0 cm in diameter

Oedema: fluid (in the skin)

Onycholysis: lifting/separation of the nail plate off the nail bed

Papule: circumscribed raised lesion of 0.5-1.0 cm in diameter

Pedunculated: lesion/mass supported on a stalk

Plaque: circumscribed elevated plateau area, usually greater than 1 cm in diameter

Pruritus: itching (a sensation you feel)

Purpura: purple non-blanching colour in the skin, usually due to damaged vasculature

Stomatitis: inflammation of the mucous lining of the oral cavity

Telangiectasia: small, dilated blood vessels near the skin/mucosal surface

Ulceration: results from loss of the entire epidermis and dermis

Vesicles: fluid-filled lesions (blister – usually clear fluid, may be haemorrhagic)

History

A 26-week-old baby boy attends your clinic with his mother. He has developed a generalized dry, red, itchy rash over the past seven weeks. His mother has been applying a regular emollient diligently and using a bath emollient. She reports that he is waking more and more frequently at night and appears to be troubled by his skin. She is worried about weaning him. He is currently breast-fed and his mother has an unrestricted diet. He has been offered a bottle of formula milk, but took only 60 mL before vomiting and developing a rash. He also developed a rash when his father kissed him, immediately after eating an egg mayonnaise sandwich.

He is the first baby of his parents; his mother had asthma in childhood and his father is allergic to shellfish. There are no pets at home. His father is a smoker. The baby was born at term by normal vaginal delivery and is vaccinated to date.

Examination

His height has reached a plateau over the past eight weeks and now rests on the 9th centile for his age. He is alert and happy, although he rubs his legs vigorously when undressed. He has generally dry skin, with widespread low-grade erythema and raised, poorly defined patches of active eczema; there are widespread excoriations (Fig. 1.1) and no clinical evidence of impetiginization. He has low-grade generalized shotty lymphadenopathy. The rest of his examination is normal.

🔍 INVESTIGATIONS

Skin prick tests

Allergen	Resulting wheal	Interpretation
Positive control	5 mm	Functioning assay
Negative control	0 mm	
Egg white	11 mm	Highly likely to be allergic
Egg yolk	4 mm	Possibly allergic
Cow's milk protein	8 mm	Highly likely to be allergic
Soya	7 mm	Highly likely to be allergic
Wheat	0 mm	Not allergic
Salmon	2 mm	Not allergic
Cod	1 mm	Not allergic
Peanut	9 mm	Highly likely to be allergic

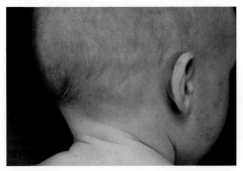

Figure 1.1

Questions

- What is this eruption?
- What associated condition does he present with?
- What dietary recommendations will you make for the baby (and mother)?

This eruption is eczema. The history his mother gives makes an associated food allergy probable – likely to egg and cow's milk protein (CMP). This, in combination with a positive family history of food allergy and asthma, means we can classify his skin condition as atopic eczema. His mother is correct to be anxious about weaning him.

It would be appropriate for this baby to be investigated for associated food allergy. Food allergy is more likely in babies presenting with eczema from a young age, and it is possible that food allergy may be contributing to the activity of his eczema and vice versa. The first line investigation should be skin prick test (SPT) to the common weaning food protein allergens (CMP, egg, soya, wheat, and fish). Peanut is commonly added to this initial panel.

The history suggests that this baby is likely to be allergic to egg and CMP, and this has been confirmed by SPT. It would be worth restricting his mother's intake of these proteins if she intends to continue breast-feeding as this may improve eczema control. If his mother wishes to stop breast-feeding, the most appropriate alternative at his age would be an amino acid formula. The incidence of coexisting CMP and soya allergy is high and the positive SPT would suggest this baby is currently allergic to both. CMP and egg are nutritionally important and ensuring a balanced diet while restricting both can be challenging; specialist dietetic advice is important. Low-grade exposure to allergenic proteins through maternal milk might be contributing to skin signs and his static growth parameters.

Regular use of topical emollients and avoidance of detergents are essential for maintaining the skin barrier function of infants with eczema. It is unlikely, however, that emollients and dietary restriction alone will suffice in the management of his eczema. His parents should be introduced to the practical aspects of topical therapy and a 'step-up, step-down' approach to the management of flares. They should be taught to identify flares early and initiate effective therapy quickly.

The association of early-onset eczema and egg allergy is associated with a three-fold increased risk of asthma in later childhood. This is an important opportunity to discuss the potential contribution paternal smoking would have on increasing that risk. Reassuringly, both egg and CMP allergy are frequently outgrown, although peanut allergy is more likely to persist.

 KEY POINTS

- Atopic eczema frequently presents within the first year of life and early onset is associated with risk of associated food allergy.
- Eczema before the age of 1 year and egg allergy are associated with an increased risk of developing asthma.
- Appropriate allergy testing and dietary advice will help prevent unsupervised dietary manipulation by well-meaning but misguided parents and may help improve eczema control.

History

A 5-year-old girl who is well known to your practice attends with her mother. She has been troubled by worsening pruritus over the last six weeks. She has missed more than ten days of school in the last month. Her mother reports that she wakes frequently at night and is lethargic and moody during the day. Her bed sheets are covered in flecks of blood in the morning.

The girl is known to be allergic to egg, fish and peanut, and has begun to develop the symptoms of seasonal allergic rhinoconjunctivitis within the last couple of months. She has a positive family history of atopy, both parents are allergic to animals and her older brother has asthma. Her younger brother has been sent home from nursery with impetigo recently.

Her treatments include an emollient as soap and leave-on preparation and various strengths of topical steroids ranging from very mild to moderately potent depending on site and eczema severity. On questioning, however, mother reports that her daughter's skin is so sore that she is refusing to bathe or apply her topical treatment.

Examination

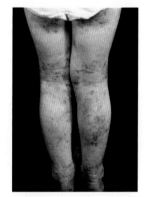

Figure 2.1

A full examination reveals a fractious child; she is unable to stop scratching her skin once undressed. She is slim, with her height at the 25th centile and weight at the 4th centile for her age. She has widespread, mildly tender, shotty lymphadenopathy (cervical, axillary and groin). Her skin is generally mildly erythrodermic and extensively excoriated, particularly her limbs (Fig. 2.1), neck and lower back. The excoriations are covered with haemorrhagic crust and yellowish exudates.

🔎 INVESTIGATIONS		
		Normal
Haemoglobin	11.2 g/dL	13.3–17.7 g/dL
Mean corpuscular volume (MCV)	87 fL	90–99 fL
White cell count	13.7 × 10⁹/L	3.9–10.6 × 10⁹/L
Platelets	498 × 10⁹/L	150–440 × 10⁹/L
Sodium	135 mmol/L	135–145 mmol/L
Potassium	4.2 mmol/L	3.5–5.0 mmol/L
Urea	5.7 mmol/L	2.5–6.7 mmol/L
Creatinine	68 mmol/L	70–120 μmol/L
Albumin	38 g/L	35–50 g/L
Bilirubin	12 mmol/L	3–17 mmol/L
Alanine transaminase	26 IU/L	5–35 IU/L
Alkaline phosphatase	238 IU/L	30–300 IU/L
Ferritin	22 ng/mL	20–200 ng/mL
Vitamin D	38 ng/mL	40–80 ng/mL

Questions

- What is the primary diagnosis?
- What secondary complications are exacerbating her pruritus?
- How would you manage this patient?

The primary diagnosis is atopic eczema associated with a positive family history of atopy as well as manifestations of IgE-mediated (immediate-type) hypersensitivity (food allergy and allergic rhinoconjunctivitis). This is clearly a moderate to severe flare of her eczema. The severity of eczema can be 'scored' by various validated subjective (e.g. CDLQI – children's dermatology life quality index) and objective scoring systems. Crudely, however, the impact on sleep and school attendance as well as the clinical severity of her eczema demonstrated in the photograph denotes severe eczema with significant functional disruption.

There may be several factors contributing to the current flare. It is likely that there is an element of secondary infection with *Staphylococcus aureus* or impetiginization of this child's eczema. The extensive yellow crusting of her excoriations, her tender lymphadenopathy, and the fact that her brother has impetigo, suggest colonization of the patient and potentially other family members. Difficulty in adhering to a bathing regime is likely to contribute. Other potential factors which worsen pruritus include iron deficiency. She is also vitamin D deficient, presumably due to her dietary restriction (egg and fish are the main dietary sources of vitamin D).

It is important to gain control of this child's eczema rapidly. Swabs should be taken for microbiology culture and sensitivity testing both from the patient and her immediate family members. As there appear to be at least two members of the family affected by *Staphylococcus aureus* it would be worthwhile considering Staphylococcus eradication protocol for the entire family (i.e. antiseptic washes and antibacterial nasal ointment). The patient might benefit from a 5–10-day course of antibiotic with good *Staphylococcus aureus* coverage (first line: flucloxacillin; second line: erythromycin or co-amoxiclav). The extensive use of a moderately potent topical corticosteroid ointment for 2–4 weeks may be required before weaning back to weak preparations or calcineurin inhibitors as maintenance therapy.

 KEY POINTS

- Atopic eczema is by definition eczema associated with a personal and/or family history of atopy.
- *Staphylococcus aureus* may cause severe flare of eczema.
- Management of such a flare includes *Staphylococcus aureus* eradication as well as appropriate treatment of the eczema.

History

A 6-year-old boy is brought to the accident and emergency department by his parents with a 5-day history of worsening eczema associated with malaise and lethargy. In addition to worsening pruritus and sleeplessness he complains of painful skin, particularly around his face, neck, chest and forearms. He quantifies the level of pain as 8 out of 10. His current flare is not responding to diligent application of his usual eczema treatments according to his 'step-up' management plan.

The onset of his eczema was at the age of 4 months, and although moderately severe in infancy it has been reasonably controlled since starting primary school, with regular use of emollients and mild to moderately potent topical steroids. His background history includes egg allergy (now partially outgrown in that he tolerates well cooked egg in cakes) and asthma, currently stable. He has never been admitted to hospital before. He is fully vaccinated to date and had chickenpox at the age of 4 years. His father suffers from hay-fever and experienced childhood eczema and asthma. He has one older sister (aged 14) who is well.

His medication includes:
- Regular emollients both as leave-on preparations and soap substitute
- Topical tacrolimus 0.1% twice daily applied to affected areas for the management of flares
- Hydroxyzine 10 mg nocte during flares and salbutamol inhaler on a prn basis

Examination

He looks unwell and is febrile at 38.5 °C. Systemic examination is normal except for widespread lymphadenopathy. There is no evidence of conjunctival erythema and his vision is normal. He has generalized moderate to severe eczema with erythema, dryness, excoriation and lichenification. He has a superimposed monomorphic eruption over his lower face, chest and forearms. The eruption is composed of multiple 23-mm monomorphic 'punched-out' erythematous lesions in various stages of evolution (Fig. 3.1). Some of the lesions are vesicular, others pustular, some coalescing, most are eroded and covered with a golden exudate and others haemorrhagic crust.

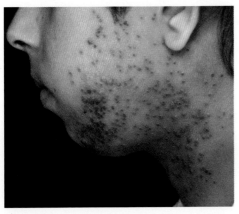

Figure 3.1

Questions
- What are these lesions?
- How would you confirm the diagnosis?
- What complications can be associated with them?
- What is their management?

These are typical lesions of herpes simplex virus (HSV) infection complicating atopic eczema. This eruption is called eczema herpeticum, or less commonly Kaposi's varicelliform eruption.

Diagnosis can be confirmed by viral swab of a blister or eroded area. Many tests can detect HSV within tissue or blister fluid. HSV can be inferred by positive staining or electron microscopy or specifically identified as types IISV-1 or HSV-2 by immunofluorescence, culture, or polymerase chain reaction. Bacteriology swab for microscopy and culture should also be undertaken.

Significant morbidity is associated with eczema herpeticum. The main potential complications include superimposed bacterial infection (Staphylococcus or Streptococcus) with risk of systemic sepsis, ocular involvement (in particular, HSV keratitis) and, rarely, systemic HSV infection with risk of spread to the liver, the lungs, the brain, the gastrointestinal tract and even the adrenal glands. In addition pain and discomfort associated with eczema herpeticum is significant.

The management of widespread eczema herpeticum includes systemic treatment of HSV infection with aciclovir, identification and treatment of any superimposed bacterial infection or strategies to prevent superimposed infection, such as antibacterial washes and creams. Topical tacrolimus should be discontinued in this patient as this may exacerbate the cutaneous spread of HSV. These cases are usually managed as in-patients, initially with intravenous aciclovir – as oral preparations can be poorly absorbed. Ophthamological review should be sought in cases of diffuse facial herpes simplex infection or where conjunctival/corneal involvement is suspected.

In a minority of cases recurrences can occur. Rapid treatment of incipient lesions with topical aciclovir may help prevent disseminated eczema herpeticum.

 KEY POINTS

- Herpes simplex infection in patients with eczema can lead to widespread lesions and an associated risk of superimposed bacterial infection and sepsis.
- It is important to consider and exclude the rare associated complication of herpes keratitis.
- In-patient management with systemic anti-viral therapy, topical antiseptic measures, pain relief, and where indicated antibiotic therapy, is required.

History

A 29-year-old man attends your clinic with a 4-year history of a recurrent and itchy facial eruption that he feels is unsightly. He notices the eruption is worse in the winter and tends to improve over the summer. He is currently studying for business exams and feels the associated stress has triggered the current flare. He avoids soaps, which make his face sore, and recently has reduced his alcohol intake in an effort to improve his eruption. He is otherwise well and on no medication.

Examination

A full examination is unremarkable except for the skin of his face, neck, central chest and scalp. There are poorly defined erythematous patches with overlying adherent greasy scale affecting his naso-labial folds and extending onto his cheeks (Fig. 4.1). His eyebrows, scalp, nape of his neck and central chest are similarly affected.

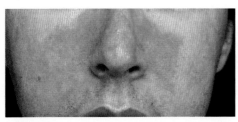

Figure 4.1

Questions

- What is this eruption?
- What age groups are affected?
- How would you manage this patient?

This eruption is seborrhoeic dermatitis. It is more common among men and typically affects the sebum-rich areas of the face, scalp and chest. The pathophysiology of seborrhoeic dermatitis is incompletely understood, however. It is linked with *Malassezia* yeast, complement activation and abnormalities of T-cell immunity. It may worsen in individuals infected with HIV or affected by Parkinson's disease.

The condition usually begins around puberty with a peak of incidence between 25 and 40 years of age. An infantile form of seborrhoeic dermatitis may manifest as cradle cap (Fig. 4.2), facial greasy scaly dermatitis, napkin dermatitis and, rarely, as an erythroderma.

In predisposed individuals seborrhoeic dermatitis usually recurs. Treatment is aimed, therefore, at reducing morbidity and preventing flares. Treatment aims are two-fold: reducing the yeast burden as a secondary preventative measure, and switching off the resultant secondary dermatitis when it occurs. Although topical corticosteroids may improve appearances of the dermatitis in the short term, they are thought to hasten recurrences and may foster dependence due to a 'rebound effect' and are usually discouraged. The use of a ketoconazole shampoo, with frequent washing and prolonged lathering often improves associated dandruff and may improve the facial involvement by depletion of *Malassezia*. Use of ketoconazole shampoo as a face wash can be irritating, but if tolerated may improve erythema and scaling. Ketoconazole or miconazole cream, calcineurin inhibitors in combination with antiseptic emollient washes are recommended. For severe or refractory seborrhoeic dermatitis systemic itraconazole as a short course or 'pulsed' (one week per month) is highly effective at reducing the yeast burden.

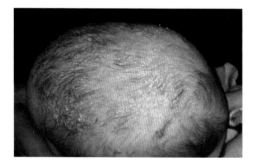

Figure 4.2

 KEY POINTS

- Seborrhoeic dermatitis is characterized by poorly defined erythematous patches with overlying greasy, yellowish-brown scale localized to the sebum-rich areas.
- It occurs most commonly among men from adolescence to middle age. Infantile seborrhoeic eczema can also occur.
- HIV infection and Parkinson's disease are both associated with refractory seborrhoeic dermatitis.

CASE 5: BLISTERED HANDS AND FEET IN AN ATHLETIC MAN

History

A 27-year-old man attends your clinic with a 3-day history of a severe burning itch over his hands associated with localized blistering and similar although less severe changes on his feet. He is otherwise well, although he did suffer from asthma is childhood and occasionally still experiences hay fever. He is on no medication. He works as a graphic designer and his hobbies include cycling and football, he has no exposure to allergens or irritants. He is unaware of any triggering factor.

Examination

He has diffuse vesicles, coalescing to form tense bullae over the palmar aspects of both hands extending into the interdigital spaces (Fig. 5.1) and onto the dorsa of his fingers and hand. In addition he has erythema, maceration, fissuring and peeling between the 4th and 5th toes on the left side and bilateral but asymmetrical (left worse than right) purulent vesicles over the insteps.

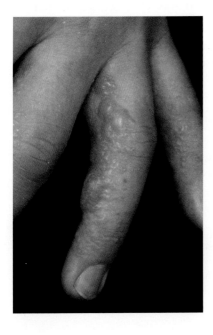

Figure 5.1

Questions

- What is the diagnosis?
- What investigations would you perform?
- What treatments would you initiate?

The diagnosis is pompholyx or dyshidrotic eczema, the symmetrical and diffuse clear vesicles over the palmar aspect of the hands associated with pruritus are highly suggestive and the diagnosis is based on clinical features. Other differential diagnoses to consider include contact dermatitis (irritant or allergic), friction blisters (e.g. epidermolysis bullosa simplex), herpes simplex infection, and palmoplantar pustular psoriasis.

Atopy appears to be a predisposing factor for pompholyx. There are several potential triggers of pompholyx including stress and as an 'id reaction' to a distant dermatophyte infection. In this case the features of interdigital maceration associated with inflammatory pustules and vesicles on the instep are suggestive of inflammatory tinea pedis.

Investigations should include scrapings from the feet (interdigital spaces and affected areas over the plantar aspects) and hands for mycological tests (direct microscopy and culture). In this case, scrapings from the feet demonstrated hyphae and spores on direct microscopy with subsequent culture confirming the presence of the zoophilic organism *Trichophyton mentagrophytes* var. *mentagrophytes*. There was no fungal infection of the hands.

Treatment of a pompholyx 'id reaction' involves treatment of the tinea pedis as well as treatment of the pompholyx itself. Inflammatory tinea pedis is usually managed with systemic antifungal therapy (itraconzole, terbinafine or fluconazole). Infected scales can be present on clothing or within footwear, so frequent laundering is recommended. Draining the larger bullae with a sterile needle will reduce the discomfort. Compresses or soaks with dilute potassium permanganate help to dry the vesicles and prevent secondary bacterial infection. Potent or superpotent topical corticosteroids are the mainstay of therapy. In the short term a combination preparation of topical corticosteroids and antibacterial agent is useful. Occasionally, systemic steroids are required.

 KEY POINTS

- Pompholyx occurs as a manifestation of hand eczema, irritant or allergic dermatitis and as an 'id reaction' to a distant dermatophyte infection.
- The mainstay of treatment is the prevention of secondary infection and use of potent or superpotent topical corticosteroids as well as identification and eradication of the trigger.

History

A 67-year-old woman presents to the vascular surgeons with varicose veins. She had a history of venous ulceration in the past, which has now healed and she is being considered for bilateral varicose vein surgery. At the consultation she complained of a 3-month history of skin itching and redness, particularly on the right lower leg, and was noted to have unilateral erythema and was referred to dermatology for an opinion.

Examination

This patient has obvious dilated and tortuous veins on both lower legs. Confluent background dull erythema is seen on the right lower leg, with small inflammatory superficial erythematous erosions and excoriations (Fig. 6.1). Palpation revealed warm, dry, rough skin at the affected site.

🔍 INVESTIGATIONS

Vascular studies
Resting pressure *right:* 174 mmHg, *left:* 180 mmHg, *brachial:* 167 mmHg
Resting ankle/brachial pressure index *right:* 1.042, *left:* 1.078. Bilateral triphasic pulsatile waveforms
Venous studies showed bilateral saphenofemoral reflux.

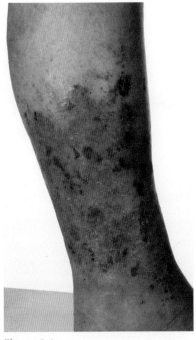

Figure 6.1

Questions

- What is the diagnosis?
- What treatment would you recommend for her right leg prior to vein surgery?
- Is this patient suitable for compression hosiery based on the vascular studies?

This patient has chronic cutaneous changes seen on the right lower leg consistent with the diagnosis of varicose eczema. This common cutaneous eruption usually has an insidious onset over many weeks to months in patients with a background of venous incompetence. The affected skin is pruritic and dry with marked erythema which may be variable in intensity depending on its chronicity. In the context of venous insufficiency, pitting oedema may develop owing to poor venous return leaving the skin tight and oedematous. This results in reduced blood flow to the skin, leading to active dusky erythema and resultant erosions or even ulceration.

Varicose eczema can be readily distinguished from cellulitis affecting the lower leg. Varicose eczema usually develops slowly, is frequently bilateral, pruritus is marked, the skin surface is rough and dry, and there are associated varicose veins. Frequently there is a background brown discolouration of the affected skin area due to haemosiderin deposition. Haemosiderin pigment is derived from haemoglobin, which is left behind in the skin when red blood cells extravasate into the tissue.

Management of the skin requires a combination of topical therapy and if possible compression. The leg should be washed with aqueous cream or an antiseptic emollient such as Dermol 500®. A moderately potent topical steroid should be applied to the eczematous areas and a rich bland emollient. Compression hosiery or two to four layer bandaging is essential to 'squeeze' the fluid out of the legs and allow skin healing. If the ankle/brachial pressure index (APBI) is above 0.8 then the arteries are sufficiently patent to permit compression without compromising the arterial blood supply to the lower extremities.

 KEY POINTS

- Varicose eczema can be distinguished from cellulitis by slow onset, pruritus and surface xerosis.
- Management of the eczema will not succeed without addressing the underlying oedema.
- Potent topical steroids should be applied to the active eczema areas plus emollients and compression.

History

A 59-year-old bus driver presents with a 5-month history of a persistent itchy patch below his umbilicus. Initially it began as an intermittent eruption, coming and going in an apparently random pattern; over the past six weeks, since the weather became warmer, it has persisted. He is otherwise well with no history of previous skin problems. He is not on medication.

Examination

There is a localized area of marked lichenification, post-inflammatory hyperpigmentation, excoriation and erosion at the midline below his umbilicus (Fig. 7.1). The surrounding skin has a more diffuse area of low-grade lichenification, hyperpigmentation and mild erythema.

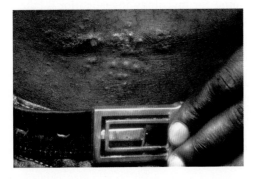

Figure 7.1

Questions

- What could this eruption be?
- How should he be investigated?
- What information does this man need?

These lesions are best described as chronic and eczematous. Such a localized problem suggests an exogenous aetiology (the photograph that is Fig. 7.1 provides a clue). The most likely diagnosis is allergic contact dermatitis (ACD), although it can be very difficult to differentiate clinically between ACD and irritant contact dermatitis. Occasionally, psoriasis may present with a single plaque, particularly at a site of trauma (Koebner's effect); however, it is rarely as pruritic as this eruption. Atopic dermatitis is usually a more generalized and diffuse eruption; however discoid or nummular eczema is characterized by fairly well defined, coin-shaped, intensely pruritic inflamed areas of lichenified skin. An inflammatory tinea corporis particularly associated with a zoophilic organism might also be considered. The presentation of contact dermatitis can be varied, including dyspigmentation, pustular lesions, urticaria, atrophy, phototoxic reactions and eczema.

It would be appropriate to obtain a skin scraping for mycology investigations. Patch testing (Fig. 7.2) is the diagnostic test to detect sensitization to contact allergens. (Although patch testing is not required for diagnosis; nickel allergy is one of the few types of allergic contact dermatitis where the history of exposure along with the signs and symptoms are quite distinctive.) In fact many patients do not present to medical practitioners as they may well work out the association themselves. If a patch test series confirms the presence of nickel allergy, its relevance to the current eruption should be confirmed. A dimethylglyoxime (DMG) test is a simple, inexpensive way to determine whether the object in question contains nickel by a pink colour change. Chromate, palladium and cobalt are commonly found together with nickel and concomitant allergy may coexist.

Nickel is a leading cause of allergic contact dermatitis and is responsible for more cases than all other metals combined. Certain occupations with high exposure to nickel, such as cashiers, hairdressers, metal workers, domestic cleaners, food handlers, bar workers, and painters, are also at risk for acquiring nickel dermatitis. Patients with atopic eczema are also at increased risk. Sweating may increase the severity of the dermatitis. Sodium chloride in the sweat causes corrosion of the metal and increases nickel exposure.

The management of this case includes removal of the offending nickel-containing belt buckle or trouser rivet and application of topical corticosteroid creams until the eruption has resolved. The patient also requires information about his allergy, that is he will always remain allergic to nickel and to both the common and unexpected sources of nickel. Nickel allergy is commonly associated with earrings and jewellery or other body piercing. Nickel can be found in many everyday items – from coins to necklace clasps, from watchbands to eyeglass frames, and tools and utensils used in the workplace and home.

Patch testing (Fig. 7.2)

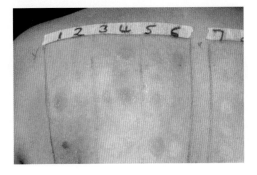

Figure 7.2 This shows an example of patch testing in a different patient. The erythematous areas over the upper back demonstrate positive eczematous reactions at day 5 of patch testing.

Day 1	*Detailed history:* Questions focus on exposures at home and work. Understand work environment. Better or worse on holidays? List of all personal care products. Hobbies and past-times.
	Choice of patch test series: The European Standard Battery (25 most common contact allergens) will identify ~80% of contact allergens. Commonly specific extended series performed according to likely exposure (e.g. healthcare series)
	Application of patch tests: Allergens applied within Finn chambers directly to upper back. Secured with adhesive tape.
Day 3 (after 48 h)	*First reading:* Patient returns. Inspect patches (ensure adequate adhesion). Mark individual sites. Score any positive reactions (+/−, 1+ to 3+ or irritant)
Day 5 (after 72 h)	*Second reading:* Score any positive reactions (as above). Interpret the results. Review exposure and product constituents. Patient information: once identified, patients are provided with written information sheets about any allergens to which they reacted.

 KEY POINTS

- Nickel is the most common allergen detected in patch test clinics worldwide. It is a strong silver-coloured metal that is commonly used in buckles, utensils and coins. It should no longer be present in jewellery purchased within the European Union.
- A useful test to confirm whether a particular item contains nickel is the dimethylglyoxime (DMG) test.
- The management includes treatment of the manifestation and avoidance of direct cutaneous contact with nickel.

History

You are asked to review a 72-year-old retired hairdresser, who attends the leg-ulcer clinic because of a 4-week history of progressive worsening pruritus of her right lower leg. Prior to this she had a venous ulcer over the medial malleolus of her right leg, which has gradually healed over a 4-month period with the diligent application of three-layer compression bandaging by her local nursing team. Her treatment regime includes a wash with chlorhexidine containing emollient lotion, application of paraffin emollient to the entire lower leg, followed by betamethasone–neomycin ointment applied directly to areas of stasis eczema and easy-release gauze over the ulcerated area. The three-layer bandages are changed twice weekly. Skin swabs have been taken over the past couple of weeks because of the worsening skin rash.

She is otherwise well. Her only oral medication is bendroflumethiazide 2.5 mg daily for hypertension.

Examination

Physical examination reveals a large but localized area of intense erythema and skin swelling confined to the anterior, posterior and medial aspect of her right lower leg (Fig. 8.1). There is marked exudate with suggestion of surface vesiculation. No involvement of her skin above her knee or foot is apparent. Although her skin is sore and itchy there is no swelling or tenderness of her calf. She has no palpable lymphadenopathy. The rest of her examination including peripheral arterial examination was normal.

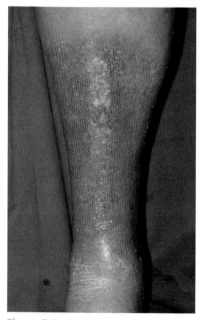

Figure 8.1

		Normal
Haemoglobin	12.8 g/dL	13.3–17.7 g/dL
Mean corpuscular volume	91 gL	80–99 fL
White cell count	45×10^9/L	$3.9–10.6 \times 10^9$/L
Platelets	196×10^9/L	$150–440 \times 10^9$/L
C-reactive protein	4	<5 mg/L
Sodium	136	135–145 mmol/L
Potassium	4.0	3.5–5.0 mmol/L
Urea	5.3	2.5–6.7 mmol/L
Creatinine	69	70–120 µmol/L
Albumin	38	35–50 g/L
Glucose	4.3	4.0–6.0 mmol/L
Bilirubin	18	3–17 mmol/L
Alanine transaminase	32	5–35 IU/L
Alkaline phosphatase	146	30–300 IU/L
Skin swab (4 and 12 days ago – identical reports)	No growth	

Questions

- What is likely to have caused the acute deterioration?
- How would you investigate this patient?
- What advice will you give the patient?

With acute erythema and swelling of the leg one of the most important differential diagnoses to consider would be a deep venous thrombosis (DVT). However DVTs are not associated with the significant degree of epidermal change seen in this case, particularly in the absence of any other suggestive features (such as swelling or intramuscular tenderness). The negative skin swab does not rule out cellulitis; the morphology and distribution of the eruption would, however, be atypical and the absence of raised white cell count or inflammatory markers effectively rules it out.

The clinical features in this case are highly suggestive of dermatitis (stasis, irritant or allergic contact dermatitis). The extensive involvement and vesiculation would be unusual for stasis dermatitis, which is usually confined to the 'gaiter' area, particularly above the medial malleolus.

The most appropriate investigation would be patch testing. Individuals with stasis dermatitis and stasis ulcers are at high risk for developing allergic contact dermatitis to topical medications applied to inflamed or ulcerated skin. Patients may also develop allergies to constituents of the bandages and dressings applied. The chronicity of this condition and the frequent occlusion of applied medications in these patients contribute to the high risk of allergic contact dermatitis to preservatives in medications and/or to the active ingredients in topical medications. Although neomycin penetrates intact skin poorly, it is an important cause of allergic contact dermatitis when applied to patients with venous stasis/ulceration. It is used surprisingly frequently despite the lack of documentation of its efficacy in the treatment of stasis ulcers. (Its poor penetration may explain the fact that a positive patch test reaction to neomycin may be delayed for four days or later following initial application.)

Individuals may develop widespread dermatitis from topical medications applied to leg ulcers or from cross-reacting systemic medications administered intravenously. Neomycin is also commonly found in combination preparations with other antibacterials and corticosteroids. These prescription and non-prescription preparations are used to treat a variety of skin, eye and external ear disorders that have become infected and inflamed. Neomycin is also present as a preservative in some vaccine preparations. It should be assumed that individuals allergic to neomycin are allergic to chemically related aminoglycoside antibiotics (e.g. gentamicin, tobramycin) and these agents should be avoided (topically or systemically).

Cross reactions with neomycin

- Framycetin
- Gentamicin
- Kanamycin
- Paromomycin
- Spectinomycin
- Streptomycin
- Tobramycin
- Co-reacts with bacitracin

KEY POINTS

- The possibility of an external cause of dermatitis must always be considered if the dermatitis is linear or sharply defined.
- Medications are important causes of allergic contact dermatitis. Individuals with stasis dermatitis are at high risk for developing allergic contact dermatitis.
- Individuals may develop allergy to preservatives in medications and/or to the active ingredients in topical medications, especially neomycin and topical corticosteroids.

History

A 26-year-old woman attends the dermatology clinic complaining of a 4-month history of an itchy eruption. She describes the eruption as 'cloud-like'. She previously suffered from eczema as a child but this rash is different. She tells you that although the eruption waxes and wanes, with individual lesions lasting 8 to 12 hours, she is rarely clear of lesions for more than half a day. Sometimes she goes to bed with the eruption and wakes clear, but the opposite can also occur. She has never experienced angioedema. She tells you it is often worse peri-menstrually. You question her about possible precipitants; she tells you that the eruption is worse with exercise or a hot bath, but does not appear to be aggravated by pressure or cold. The eruption is partially attenuated by cetirizine 10 mg daily, which she is taking for her hayfever. Her only other medication is occasional ibuprofen for dysmenorrhoea.

There is no family history of skin lesions. Both of her parents are well, although her mother has a diagnosis of osteoporosis and is on thyroxine replacement. On close questioning she admits that although circumstances at work are stable and have not changed for a longtime she is experiencing difficulty coping and frequently cries at work.

Examination

On examination there are several scattered lesions over her trunk, limbs and face. They are composed of well-defined erythematous oedematous plaques surrounded by a pale 'flare' (Fig. 9.1). The lesions vary in size and shape but not in morphology. You are unable to elicit dermographism. The lesion that you ringed initially had disappeared by the time she presented to photography 2 hours later, with new lesions developing over adjacent skin.

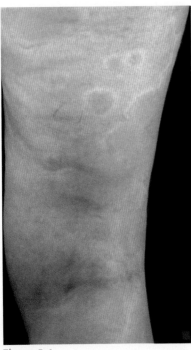

Figure 9.1

Following their resolution the lesions leave no persistent skin change. Although the eruption is pruritic there is no evidence of lichenification or excoriations. Her blood pressure is 105/68 mmHg and pulse rate 102 beats/min. Examination of her cardiorespiratory system is otherwise normal. Her abdomen is soft and non-tender. You notice a degree of bilateral upper eyelid lag. She has a smoothly enlarged goitre and stretching her hands out she has a fine tremor.

Examination of the remainder of the neurological system is normal. Urinalysis was negative for blood, white cells and glucose. You ask the patient to put on her coat and walk briskly up and down the corridor outside. After five minutes she returns with a marked aggravation of her eruption, which is now widespread and generalized over her trunk and proximal limbs. You draw around a well-defined skin lesion and request some further investigations.

Full blood count	Normal
Urea and electrolytes	Normal
Liver function tests	Normal

Questions

- What is this eruption?
- What factors in the history and on examination might be contributing to the eruption?
- How would you investigate this patient?
- What is the management?

This patient is suffering from urticaria, which is characterized by wheals or 'hives' that represent areas of cutaneous mast cell degranulation, releasing histamine and other mediators, followed by transient oedema and erythema. When urticaria persists for more than 6 weeks it is classified as chronic urticaria. It represents a tissue reaction pattern and can be precipitated by a variety of stimuli or triggers. Many skin eruptions are known which may present with 'urticated' lesions that are not transient.

There may be more than one precipitant of urticaria in any one affected individual. Although there is an element of physical provocation, which you have demonstrated by exercising the patient, the eruption can be present on waking and therefore there is more to this than cholinergic urticaria. The patient is atopic, a factor reported to be associated with urticaria. She has made an interesting observation that her urticaria is worse peri-menstrually; the phenomenon of progesterone-provoked urticaria is described. It is more likely, however, that the exacerbation is due to her use of a non-steroidal anti-inflammatory drug (ibuprofen). Importantly, she has clinical features of thyrotoxicosis – chronic urticaria is associated with a number of autoimmune diseases, particularly autoimmune thyroid disease (Graves' disease), systemic lupus erythmatosus (SLE) and cryoglobulinaemia.

Urticarial vasculitis is an important differential diagnosis of chronic urticaria. Typically the lesions of urticarial vasculitis are associated with a burning pain and persist for more than 24 hours. They may leave post-inflammatory hyperpigmentation or ecchymoses on resolution and can be diagnosed by the demonstration of a leucocytoclastic vasculitis on biopsy of affected skin. Where urticarial vasculitis is suspected a work-up for potential systemic vasculitis is important.

The initial investigation of this patient would include complete blood cell count, erythrocyte sedimentation rate, thyroid function tests, antithyroid antibodies (antithyroid microsomal and peroxidase antibodies), basophil histamine release assay. Other tests which might be considered: skin biopsy, antinuclear antibodies (ANA), C3, C4 (if features of urticarial vasculitis or associated angioedema suggesting acquired C1 esterase deficiency secondary to SLE), cryoglobulins and cryoprecipitans (if history of cold-induced urticaria).

It is clear that this patient has symptomatic thyrotoxicosis, so its management and control may significantly improve or even resolve her urticaria. In the short term propranolol may be indicated until carbimazole achieves a euthyroid state. For any persisting urticaria non-sedating antihistamines (anti-H1) are the mainstay of treatment. Response to different antihistamines can vary so it may be worthwhile trialling different agents, and in some cases doses higher than those required in allergic rhinoconjunctivitis may be needed. The addition of anti-H2 antihistamine such as ranitidine or cimetidine may provide some additional blockade of histamine receptors and can be beneficial, as can the addition of a leukotriene receptor antagonist such as montelukast. In general these agents are well tolerated. For patients with evidence of autoimmune association and troublesome persistent urticaria, immunosuppressive therapy with agents such as ciclosporin or methotrexate may be required.

Causes of chronic urticaria

- *Medication:* Aspirin, other nonsteroidal anti-inflammatory drugs, opioids, ACE inhibitors, radiological contrast media.
- *Physical urticaria:* The most common causes of urticaria frequently coexist:
  - Dermatographism/dermographism – firm stroking
  - Delayed pressure urticaria – pressure (6–24 h after the application of pressure)
  - Cold urticaria – the cold
  - Aquagenic urticaria – water exposure
  - Cholinergic urticaria – heat, exercise or stress
  - Solar urticaria – sun exposure
  - Vibratory urticaria – vibration

- *Autoimmune disease:* Autoimmune thyroid disease, systemic lupus erythematosus, cryoglobulinaemia.
- *Autoimmune urticaria:* Immunoglobulin G autoantibodies to alpha subunit of the Fc receptor of the immunoglobulin E (IgE) molecule (35–40 per cent) or, less commonly, anti-IgE autoantibodies (5–10 per cent), can activate basophils to release histamine, the basis of an in-vitro basophil histamine release assay. Autoimmune urticaria is closely associated with positive anti-thyroid antibodies.
- *Viral infections* are the most common cause of chronic urticaria in children.
- *Foods and food additives:* Some patients report the exacerbation of urticaria associated with the consumption of certain foods, such as spiced food, strawberries, tinned or preserved food, or certain baked goods. Some of these foods contain natural salicylates or other chemical capable of histamine release. This reaction is distinct from IgE-mediated type I hypersensitivity to foods, which can be associated with acute urticaria.
- *Contactants:* The onset of localized (or even generalized) urticaria within 30 to 60 minutes of contact with an inciting agent such as latex (especially in health care workers), plants, animals (e.g. caterpillars, dander), medications, and food (e.g. fish, garlic, onions, tomato).
- *Autoinflammatory syndromes:* There are rare causes of urticaria such as Muckle–Wells syndrome (amyloidosis, nerve deafness, and urticaria) and Schnitzler's syndrome (fever, joint/bone pain, monoclonal gammopathy, and urticaria).
- *Idiopathic urticaria* is the descriptive term for chronic urticaria for which no precipitant can be identified.

KEY POINTS

- Urticaria is a cutaneous reaction pattern characterized by the degranulation of mast cells and transient wheals.
- There are a number of potential precipitants, exacerbating factors and underlying causes of chronic urticaria.
- The mainstay of therapy is to correct any underlying medical disorders and the use of non-sedating anti-H1 antihistamines.

History

A 16-month-old boy presents to the dermatology clinic. His mother has noticed a gradual accumulation of 'brown spots' on his skin. These lesions were not present at birth and the majority appeared as a crop over a 4-month period around his first birthday. She feels it is possible that he will continue to acquire new lesions. He had one on his right forearm which has resolved. She has noticed that some of the lesions appear to 'blister' or become raised after a bath. He is otherwise well; he is thriving and enjoys a full diet. He has no gastrointestinal symptoms or wheeze. There is no family history of similar skin lesions. The rest of the family is entirely well.

Examination

His height and weight are on the 75th and 91st centiles for his age, respectively. He is cooperative and follows directions. He has diffuse, scattered, monomorphic, small oval-round reddish-brown macules concentrated predominantly over his anterior and posterior trunk, but also extending to his neck and with a few scattered lesions on his limbs. There are more than 40 of these lesions. One lesion just below his xiphisternum, when rubbed, became transiently erythematous and swollen (urticaria), a positive Darier's sign (Fig. 10.1). Examination of his cardiorespiratory system and abdomen is normal. He has no lymphadenopathy.

INVESTIGATIONS		
		Normal
Haemoglobin	12.9 g/dL	13.3–17.7 g/dL
Mean corpuscular volume	92 fL	90–99 fL
White cell count	4.8 × 10⁹/L	3.9–10.6 × 10⁹/L
Platelets	275 × 10⁹/L	150–440 × 10⁹/L
Blood film	Normal morphology	
Sodium	138 mmol/L	135–145 mmol/L
Potassium	4.0 mmol/L	3.5–5.0 mmol/L
Urea	5.6 mmol/L	2.5–6.7 mmol/L
Creatinine	76 µmol/L	70–120 µmol/L
Albumin	38 g/L	35–50 g/L
Bilirubin	9 mmol/L	3–17 mmol/L
Alanine transaminase	14 IU/L	5–35 IU/L
Alkaline phosphatase	90 IU/L	30–300 IU/L
Tryptase	5 ng/L	< 20 ng/L

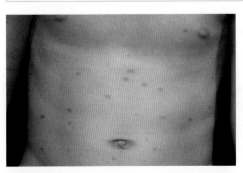

Figure 10.1

Questions

- What are these lesions?
- Would you perform any further investigations?
- What is their management?

These lesions represent multiple mastocytomas and the eruption is referred to as urticaria pigmentosa. Darier's sign describes the development of a wheal and surrounding erythema in a lesion after rubbing (physical degranulation of histamine from mast cells). Mastocytosis is the abnormal accumulation of mast cells within the skin and rarely other organs (liver, spleen or lymph nodes). The differential diagnosis would include lentigines or melanocytic naevi (if Darier's sign negative) or xanthogranuloma, histiocytosis X or generalized eruptive histiocytoma (if the lesions were raised or indurated).

All forms of mastocytosis in children have a good prognosis and systemic involvement is rare. The majority of cases resolve spontaneously. In adults, however, systemic involvement may be aggressive or even represent a mast cell leukaemia. Symptoms of systemic involvement or of acute degranulation of widespread cutaneous disease include flushing, diarrhoea, nausea/vomiting, abdominal cramps and wheeze. Adults may also complain of syncope, angina, headaches and bone pain.

Although this young patient has no symptoms of systemic disease, basic investigations would be justified including particularly full blood count, serum tryptase and liver function tests. A skin biopsy can be performed if there is diagnostic doubt. Mast cell infiltrates can be difficult to identify by routine haematoxylin & eosin staining, and special stains such as Giemsa or toluidine blue, which demonstrate metaochromatic staining of mast cells, are required. For patients with rapidly progressive disease and abnormalities of the above investigations, further testing such as bone marrow aspirate and biopsy under the supervision of the haematology department may be indicated. Demonstration of activating mutations of the c-kit proto-oncogene would help tailor therapy in aggressive or leukaemic disease (e.g. imatinib).

As the skin lesions are likely to resolve spontaneously by the boy's 10th birthday, no treatment is indicated. For patients with skin symptoms antihistamines (H1-blocker) may be helpful. Moderate sunlight exposure can hasten the resolution of diffuse lesions and psoralen–UVA can be offered to adults/older children. Patients with numerous lesions or diffuse disease should avoid mast cell degranulating agents such as non-steroidal anti-inflammatory drugs, opiates, alcohol, caffeine, radiological contrast media and abrupt physical degranulation such as a hot bath or other acute temperature change, vigorous rubbing (e.g. after a bath or by tight clothing). Exposure to degranulating agents or to allergens (such as hymenoptera stings) can potentially provoke anaphylaxis.

 KEY POINTS

- Urticaria pigmentosa is characterized by mast cell proliferation and accumulation within the skin.
- When a urticaria pigmentosa or mastocytoma lesion is stroked, it typically urticates, becoming pruritic, oedematous and erythematous. This change is referred to as Darier's sign.
- Most patients with urticaria pigmentosa exhibit onset before age 2 years. The disease is associated with an excellent prognosis, often with resolution by puberty. The number of lesions diminishes by approximately 10 per cent a year.

History

A 51-year-old man is referred for an urgent opinion with an 8-week history of intermittent swellings affecting his hands, feet, face and genitalia. He also describes intermittent abdominal bloating and pain. Over the last three weeks he had attended the accident and emergency department on two occasions. The first time, when he presented with lip and tongue swelling but without shortness of breath, he was treated with antihistamines and intravenous hydrocortisone, but did not require adrenaline or intubation. On the second occasion, with acute and severe abdominal pain associated with vomiting, he was admitted for 24 hours under the surgical team for investigation of an acute abdomen, before his symptoms spontaneously resolved. He does not describe any associated urticaria but does complain of recent-onset night sweats, weight loss and low energy levels. He is unaware of provoking factors and feels there is no pattern to the swellings as they can occur at any time including overnight.

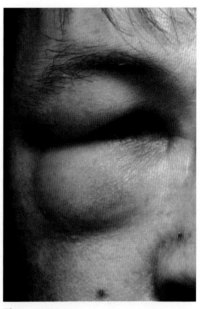

He has no previous history of atopy and is on no medication (he denies taking any over-the-counter preparations such as non-steroidal anti-inflammatory drugs). He has no family history of swellings or skin rashes. He is a non-smoker and works as a truck driver.

Examination

His skin is normal except for the presence of unilateral left-sided peri-orbital soft tissue swelling (Fig. 11.1). He has smooth, non-tender bilateral axillary and left-sided inguinal lymphadenopathy. The remainder of his examination is normal.

Figure 11.1

INVESTIGATIONS		
		Normal
Haemoglobin	10.4 g/dL	13.3–17.7 g/dL
Mean corpuscular volume	85 fL	90–99 fL
White cell count	5.6×10^9/L	$3.9–10.6 \times 10^9$/L
Platelets	132×10^9/L	$150–440 \times 10^9$/L
Urea and electrolytes	Normal	
Liver function tests	Normal	
Complement C3	53 mg/dL	75–135 mg/dL
Complement C4	5 mg/dL	12–72 mg/dL

Questions

- What are these intermittent swellings?
- What are the possible underlying diagnoses?
- How would you investigate further?

The skin swellings are angioedema. Unusually in this case angioedema is occurring in the absence of urticaria. Immunoglobulin E (IgE)-mediated allergic angioedema (provoked by food, drugs, insect bites or latex) or angioedema provoked by physical stimuli (such as sun, heat or cold) is mediated by local release of histamine and is frequently associated with hives or urticaria. The striking other clinical features in this case include the night sweats, weight loss and lymphadenopathy. He has anaemia and thrombocytopenia. The low complement levels should trigger testing of C-1 esterase inhibitor (C1-INH) levels (suggesting acquired C1-esterase inhibitor deficiency). This patient needs thorough haematological assessment looking for an underlying lymphoproliferative disorder. Further investigations include tests for serum lactate dehydrogenase and β2-microglobulin, immunoglobulins and protein electrophoresis, CT of the chest, abdomen and pelvis as well as lymph node and bone marrow biopsy.

When confronted with angioedema in the absence of urticaria it is important to consider diseases mediated by bradykinin such as C1-INH deficiency (which can be genetic or acquired) or induced by angiotensin converting enzyme (ACE) inhibitors. Hereditary angioedema is autosomal dominantly inherited, and although there is a high incidence of de-novo mutations (25 per cent), it usually presents peri-puberty or following surgery/trauma, making it a less likely diagnosis in this case. Acquired angioedema can be associated with underlying connective tissue disease (systemic lupus erythmatosus, lupus anticoagulant) or lymphoproliferative (particularly B-cell lymphoma) disorders.

Common to all of these disorders are symptoms of angioedema, in the absence of urticaria, which can include laryngeal oedema or tongue and/or pharyngeal oedema of sufficient severity as to cause airway obstruction and, potentially, asphyxia. These bradykinin-dependent disorders can also include gastrointestinal symptoms reminiscent of an acute abdomen with severe pain, nausea, vomiting, or diarrhoea due to oedema of the bowel wall. Hypotension is frequently a feature.

The management of acquired angioedema includes the use of androgens (such as danazol or stanozolol) and antifibrinolytics (such as tranexamic acid) as prophylaxis. The emphasis however is on diagnosis and treatment of the underlying disease. For hereditary angioedema, C1-INH concentrate (extracted from human plasma and freeze dried) is available for intravenous administration.

Differential diagnosis of angioedema in the absence of urticaria

- IgE mediated allergy (e.g. food, latex, drugs)
- Non-IgE mediated histamine release (e.g. physical stimuli, drugs)
- Bradykinin mediated:
  - Hereditary C1-INH deficiency
  - Acquired C1-INH deficiency (associated with lymphoproliferative or connective tissue disorders).
  - ACE inhibitors

KEY POINTS

- Angioedema in the absence of urticaria is unusual and points towards a bradykinin-mediated mechanism, most commonly C1–INH deficiency, either hereditary or acquired.
- Symptoms may include angioedema of the face, extremities and genitalia, abdominal pain and bloating, hypotension and potentially laryngeal oedema leading to asphyxiation.
- Underlying autoimmune connective tissue disease or B-cell lymphoproliferative disorders may underlie acquired angioedema.

History

A 25-year-old man presents with a rash on his knees. This had gradually worsened over three years. In addition he had previously had dandruff and more recently noticed his nails changing, for which his GP treated him for a fungal nail infection, but with no improvement. He is a smoker and drinks 35 units of alcohol per week. He has noticed an improvement during the summer months and has also developed pains in his elbow and knees. His sister had a similar rash over her elbows.

Examination

There are erythematous plaques on his knees with clearly defined borders and overlying thick scale (Fig. 12.1). There is fine scale throughout the scalp and in his external auditory canals. Examination of his finger nails reveal three nail plates with pitting and onycholysis.

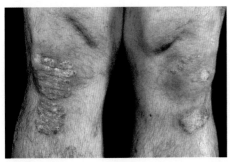

Figure 12.1

Questions

- What is the diagnosis?
- What are the risk factors for the disease?
- Are his joint pains relevant?

Clinically this patient has chronic plaque psoriasis. This is a chronic inflammatory disease that affects 2 per cent of the population. It affects not only the skin, but can also affect the nails and joints. Psoriasis can present in several different ways, but chronic plaque psoriasis is characterized by well demarcated erythematous plaques which have an overlying silvery scale that frequently affects the extensor aspects of the elbows and knees, as in this patient. Differential diagnoses of chronic plaque psoriasis include discoid eczema, tinea corporis, lichen simplex and mycosis fungoides (T-cell lymphoma).

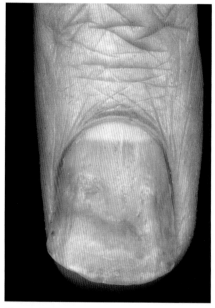

Risk factors for psoriasis include a positive family history. In addition, possible triggering and exacerbating factors include stress, smoking, alcohol, streptococcal infection and medications such as β-blockers and non-steroidal anti-inflammatory drugs (NSAIDs). Physical trauma can be a major factor in triggering lesions, the so-called Koebner phenomenon.

Nail disease in psoriasis is common, affecting the fingernails and toenails. Nail changes (Fig. 12.2) include pitting and onycholysis (separation of the nail plate from the nail bed), and subungal hyperkeratosis. Oil spots are pathognomic and appear as yellow-brown spots under the nail plate. Basic histopathology shows there is marked thickening of the epidermis (plaques) and dilated blood vessels just beneath the epidermis (erythema), and neutrophils infiltrate up into the stratum corneum where they form microabscesses of Munro (inflammation).

Figure 12.2

The different clinical presentations of psoriasis include guttate, pustular, erythrodermic and palmoplantar. It is thought that 5–10 per cent of patients with psoriasis have joint involvement known as psoriatic arthritis, which may precede, present with, or most commonly follow, the skin involvement. There are five different clinical types: asymmetric (mono– or oligoarthropathy), symmetrical polyarthritis (rheumatoid arthritis-like), distal interphalangeal joint disease, arthritis mutilans, and ankylosing-spondylitis–like.

Chronic plaque psoriasis can be treated with topical therapy including emollients, steroid ointments, vitamin-D analogues, coal tar-based preparations, dithranol, salicylic acid and phototherapy. Joint disease may respond to NSAIDs, methotrexate or ciclosporin.

Systemic drugs are reserved for moderate-to-severe recalcitrant disease and include ciclosporin, methotrexate, acitretin and in more recent years the biologics that include the biologics such as infliximab, which has anti-tumour necrosis factor activity.

 KEY POINTS

- Psoriasis is a chronic inflammatory disease affecting 2 per cent of the population.
- It affects not only the skin but can also affect the nails and joints.
- There are multiple modalities of treatments including topical, phototherapeutic and systemic drug preparations.

History

An 18-year-old girl develops a widespread rash 5 days after a sore throat. She had presented in a similar way 2 years ago to her GP who treated her with antibiotics and the rash had faded. She does not feel unwell in herself and has no other symptoms.

Examination

There are multiple erythematous small discrete plaques and papules with overlying scale predominantly over her trunk but also affecting her limbs (Fig. 13.1). Her face and scalp have been spared. Her nails are normal. Examination of her throat reveals some erythema over her pharynx, but no pustules are seen.

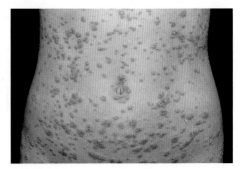

Figure 13.1

🔎 INVESTIGATIONS

Throat swab: group A β-haemolytic Streptococcus

Questions

- What is the most likely diagnosis?
- How would you manage her?
- What is the prognosis?

This patient is suffering from guttate psoriasis. This is a scaly skin eruption that appears rapidly after the onset of a streptococcal throat infection. This type of psoriasis is predominantly seen in adolescents and young adults. The word guttate is derived from the Latin name gutta which means 'drop-like'. The differential diagnosis includes *Pityriasis rosea*.

Classically, in guttate psoriasis lesions are symmetrical mainly over the trunk and limbs with crops of papules and small plaques with overlying scale. Throat swabs may confirm the presence of group A β-haemolytic Streptococcus. Blood tests may reveal an increased antistreptolysin titre.

Patients with guttate psoriasis respond well to phototherapy. Mild topical steroid can be used but it is challenging to apply the medicated ointment accurately to the affected skin only. As a general rule thin plaques of psoriasis respond well to ultraviolet B (UVB) light and thicker plaques respond to UVA light given with oral psoralen (PUVA).

This patient's throat swab confirmed a streptococcal infection and she was therefore treated with 10 days of erythromycin antibiotics. It is thought that treating the underlying bacterial infection can shorten the length of the skin eruption. Her skin cleared with narrow-band UVB phototherapy (TL-01) given three times per week for 4 weeks.

Occasionally, guttate psoriasis can evolve in some patients into chronic plaque psoriasis, many of whom have a positive family history of psoriasis. The majority of patients, however, are clear of the lesions after a few weeks. Patients may have recurrent 'attacks' associated with bacterial throat infections, as in this case.

 KEY POINTS

- Guttate psoriasis often is associated with a preceding streptococcal throat infection.
- It is predominantly seen in adolescents and young adults.
- Patients with guttate psoriasis respond well to phototherapy.

History

A 50-year-old man presents to the on-call dermatologist with a 3-day history of rigors, feeling generally unwell and redness of all his skin associated with scaling. He also complains of swelling of his arms and legs. Since his teenage years he has suffered with a scaly scalp and occasional dry patches on the elbows. There is a family history of psoriasis. Recently he has been experiencing increasing episodes of angina and has sought medical attention.

Examination

There is widespread erythema affecting the face, trunk and limbs with thickening of the skin and associated widespread scale (Fig. 14.1). Thick scale is present throughout the scalp with dystrophy of all 20 nails. Over the elbows erythematous plaques with overlying thick scale are seen. In addition there are mild bilateral ectropions.

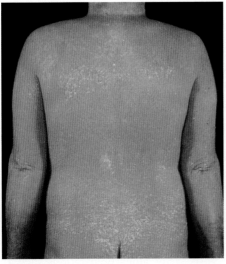

Figure 14.1

Questions

- What is the likely diagnosis?
- What is the differential diagnosis?
- How would you manage this patient?
- What are the potential complications?

The most likely diagnosis is erythrodermic psoriasis. Erythroderma is when almost the entire skin (> 90%) becomes red; in the case of psoriasis the skin is also thickened and scaly. There is usually hyperkeratosis of the palmar/plantar sites. There may be onycholysis (lifting of the nail plates) and even shedding of the nails. Thinning of the hair and alopecia may also occur. Clues in this patient to the underlying cause of his erythroderma are his dystrophic nails and classic plaques of psoriasis over his elbows. In addition he has a history of scalp scaling and a family history of psoriasis.

Erythrodema is a serious and at times life-threatening dermatological emergency. Erythrodermic skin is associated with fever, rigors and lymphadenopathy.

Other causes of erythroderma include atopic eczema, drug eruptions, cutaneous T-cell lymphoma, allergic contact dermatitis, pityriasis rubra pilaris and seborrhoeic dermatitis. To diagnose the underlying cause can be very challenging and signs and symptoms of pre-existing dermatoses may help, as in this case.

Complications result from significant physiological and metabolic changes that occur when the skin barrier function starts to fail. Thermoregulatory control is lost, leaving patients vulnerable to hypothermia due to excess heat loss. Dehydration commonly occurs owing to increased transepidermal water. Cutaneous inflammation may mask concurrent secondary skin infection and blood cultures may be positive owing to their easy contamination with normal skin flora. Hypoalbuminaemia and cardiac failure are serious complications that particularly affect the elderly.

Treatment is supportive. In-patient management and skilled nursing care are essential. Close monitoring of pulse, blood pressure, temperature and fluid balance is mandatory. Hourly emollient therapy with liquid paraffin and mild topical steroids are the mainstay of the acute phase. The use of systemic corticosteroids in the acute setting is controversial, as there is some evidence they can exacerbate the condition and may even have been the initial trigger. Adequate nutritional support to minimize protein losses is important. Haemodynamic instability and intercurrent infections are treated as necessary.

Patients usually require systemic therapy; historically ciclosporin has been given for its fast mode of action. However, some dermatologists are now treating these very sick patients with first-line systemic anti-tumour necrosis factor alpha preparations such as infliximab.

 KEY POINTS

- Erythroderma is when almost the entire skin (> 90%) becomes red.
- It is a serious and at times life-threatening dermatological emergency.
- Management is supportive in addition to treatment of the underlying cause.

History

A 20-year-old girl develops a rash 24 hours after commencing her holiday in the sun. The rash is itchy and red affecting her neck and forearms, there is sparing of her face and hands. The rash persists for approximately one week before settling with no scarring. She has no previous history of skin problems, although her mother had suffered a similar rash whilst on a sunny holiday.

Examination

There are clusters of confluent erythematous urticated papules and plaques on her neck (Fig. 15.1) and the extensor aspects of her arms. The rest of the skin is clear.

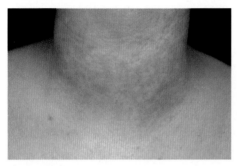

Figure 15.1

Questions

- What is the diagnosis?
- How would you manage this patient in the short/long term?

This patient has polymorphic light eruption (PLE) or 'prickly heat'. This is a very common recurring photodermatosis of unknown aetiology. It is more commonly seen in women and occurs usually about 24 hours after sun exposure as in this case. The pruritic eruption usually persists for 7–10 days. It is characterized by a polymorphous rash that can include erythematous macules, patches, papules, plaques, and sometimes vesicles and bullae. These typically affect the extensor forearms and 'V area' of the neck. The eruption classically spares the face, as in our patient.

The onset of PLE usually starts in the first three decades of life and then usually occurs each spring or early summer thereafter. Many patients improve by the end of the summer but the rash occurs the following spring or following a 'winter sun' holiday. The degree of severity is variable. There is sometimes a family history of photosensitivity.

PLE is a clinical diagnosis based on the history and it is therefore important to exclude other causes of photosensitive dermatoses such as photoallergic contact dermatitis, photo drug eruptions and lupus erythematosus. A skin biopsy can be helpful if there is any doubt.

Topical steroids are the mainstay of treatment for patients presenting with the pruritic eruption of PLE. A short course of systemic corticosteroids may be required for severe attacks. Patients should be advised to protect themselves from the sun by wearing a shirt with long sleeves. Sunscreens with high factor ultraviolet (UV) A and UVB filters can be helpful in some patients. Some patients benefit from prophylactic phototherapy (narrow-band UVB) given before the onset of spring to 'harden' the skin and thus prevent PLE when sunlight becomes more intense.

 KEY POINTS

- PLE or 'prickly heat' is a common eruption occurring during the spring or early summer.
- It occurs usually 24 hours after sun exposure and persists for 7–10 days.
- Other photodermatoses should be excluded in the first instance.

History

A 33-year-old woman presents with a sudden-onset blistering rash on her legs. On closer questioning she reports no recent history of travel or contact with animals. She recently moved into new accommodation and has been clearing an overgrown garden over the past few days. She has been clearing weeds by hand but wore garden gloves and borrowed a strimmer from a friend to cut through long grass. She felt an intense itching on her lower legs and then noticed blisters in a streaking pattern. She has no previous history of skin disease or atopy and is otherwise well.

Examination

Linear vesicular lesions with associated erythema and excoriations are seen on her legs (Fig. 16.1). There are tense bullae filled with clear serous fluid. Full skin examination is otherwise unremarkable including mucosal membranes.

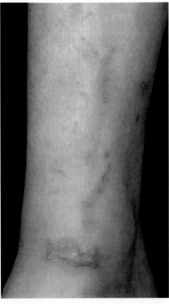

Figure 16.1

Questions

- What is the most likely diagnosis?
- What is the underlying cause?
- How would you manage this patient?

This patient is suffering from phytophotodermatitis, which is a phototoxic skin eruption. This acute inflammatory condition is triggered by the combination of skin contact with photosensitizing chemicals in plants plus sunlight. Patients usually report burning or itching of their skin prior to the onset of blistering. The characteristic skin patterns result from the plant brushing against bare skin whilst outdoors.

The diagnosis is made on the history of plant exposure and from the clinical appearance of linear blisters, usually on exposed skin. The morphology of the rash looks very exogenous (linear or bizarre-shaped streaks) with erythema, vesicles, bullae and oedema which classically resolve leaving post-inflammatory hyperpigmentation. Although gardeners are most commonly affected, exposure to lime-juice in the preparation of drinks outdoors is another typical presentation.

Phytophotodermatitis usually occurs in the spring and summer months. The main photosensitizing substances found in plants are called furocoumarins, which consist of psoralens, 5,8-methoxypsoralens, angelicin, bergaptol and xanthotal. The most common plant family implicated is the Umbelliferae, which includes giant hogweed, celery, wild parsnip and parsley. Other plant families that cause phytophotodermatitis are Rutaceae (lime) and Leguminosae (beans).

The characteristic rash may appear within minutes to hours after exposure to the plant and utraviolet light, but more usually erupts 24 hours (peak 48–72 hours) after exposure.

Phytophotodermatitis is a self-limiting skin eruption; however, it is intensely itchy and blistering. Super-potent topical steroid should be applied twice daily to the affected area for 1–2 weeks. Large tense bullae should be deflated with a sterile needle. Advice should be given to patients concerning the use of personal protective clothing if continuing with similar outdoor work.

 KEY POINTS

- Phytophotodermatitis occurs due to the combination of skin contact with photosensitizing chemicals in plants plus sunlight.
- The main photosensitizing substances found in plants are called furocoumarins.
- The acute eruption should respond to potent topical steroids.

History

A 49-year-old man presents to the dermatology out-patient clinic with a 6-month his-tory of a gradually worsening rash on the dorsi of his hands. He had first noticed a few small blisters developing in the early spring and since then more have appeared. He is concerned about the scarring marks left on his hands. He has recently been made redun-dant and as a result has been drinking large quantities of alcohol. He has no history of previous skin problems or atopy. He is otherwise well and does not take any regular medication.

Examination

Over the dorsi of his hands are scattered tense vesicles and bullae with multiple erosions, scarring, milia and pigmentation (Fig. 17.1). Full skin examination reveals similar small scars on his face and minimal hypertrichosis. The rest of the skin is normal.

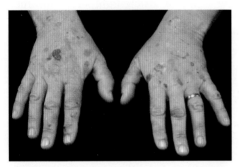

Questions

- What is the diagnosis?
- What is the underlying cause?
- How would you confirm the diagnosis?

Figure 17.1

This patient was not aware that he was photosensitive due to the insidious onset of his skin eruption over many months. Medical practitioners should suspect photosensitivity if skin disease affects exposed skin sites – classically the face, hands and anterior chest. On direct questioning, patients may report a worsening of their skin condition during the summer or following a holiday abroad.

This patient was diagnosed with porphyria cutanea tarda (PCT) which usually presents between the 3rd to 5th decades. The condition is characterized by skin fragility leading to blister formation following minor trauma. Initially, skin changes include tense vesicles/bullae and erosions on a background of normal-looking skin. However, these heal to leave small atrophic scars and milia (inclusion cysts) as seen in this patient. Waxy-looking plaques and hypertrichosis may also be seen.

Porphyrins are important in the formation of haemoglobin, myoglobin and cytochromes. The porphyrias are diseases in which specific enzyme deficiencies lead to the accumulation of intermediate metabolites in the porphyrin biosynthesis pathway. Porphyrins absorb light in the 400–405 nm range (the lower range of visible light). This absorbed light is then transferred to cellular structures, causing damage to tissues. Deficiency of the enzyme uroporphyrinogen decarboxylase (UROD) is responsible for PCT, which may be inherited or acquired. Patients with acquired disease are deficient in UROD in their liver and therefore express the disease phenotypically when triggered by agents such as alcohol, oestrogen and hepatitis C. Familial PCT is inherited in an autosomal dominant fashion with a resultant defect in the synthesis of UROD.

A skin biopsy reveals subepidermal bullae. Wood's lamp examination of the urine shows orange red fluorescence. A porphyrin screen reveals raised uroporphyrin I in the urine and increased levels of isocoproporphyrins in the stool.

Treatments include eliminating possible trigger factors such as alcohol. Patients should be protected from both ultraviolet and visible light. Management includes venesection to reduce iron stores or low-dose oral chloroquine/hydroxychloroquine.

 KEY POINTS

- PCT occurs due to deficiency of the enzyme uroporphyrinogen decarboxylase.
- It may be inherited or acquired. Triggers include alcohol, oestrogen and hepatitis C.
- Skin changes include fragility, tense vesicles/bullae, erosions, atrophic scars and milia.

History

A 16-year-old boy with scarring over his face is referred to the dermatology out-patient clinic. He reports a history of burning and stinging of his skin (especially his nose) whilst outside playing football. On direct questioning his parents recall as a small child he would cry after a few minutes of sun exposure. His parents had also noted his skin would then turn red and blister. Consequently, as a young child they tried to keep him out of the sun as much as possible. However, as a teenager keen on sports he has recently noticed a deterioration of the skin on his face. He is otherwise well and takes no medication.

Examination

Over his cheeks and nose the skin appears waxy and atrophic with multiple areas of pitted scarring (Fig.18.1). Areas of hyperpigmentation and milia are seen on the dorsal aspects of his hands.

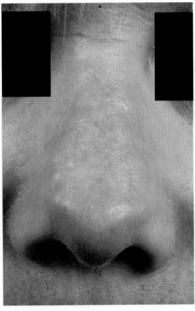

Figure 18.1

Questions

- What is the underlying diagnosis?
- How might you confirm this?
- What other diseases may be associated?

This patient has erythropoietic protoporphyria (EPP) which is a rare, hereditary autosomal-dominant metabolic disorder of porphyrin metabolism. Patients usually report symptoms starting in early childhood. Photosensitivity may be severe with almost immediate stinging, burning and itching following sun exposure. Erythema, oedema, vesicles and purpura appear within 1–8 hours predominantly over the nose, cheeks and dorsi of the hands. Similar symptoms can occur when a person is exposed to sunlight through window glass.

Over time these areas develop into shallow, atrophic and often linear scars. Diffuse wrinkling of the skin on the nose, cheeks and perioral area can also occur leaving a waxy appearance. The skin over the metacarpal phalangeal joints can become indurated and shiny ('aged knuckles').

EPP results from a deficiency in the enzyme ferrochelatase. This defect occurs at the step in porphyrin metabolism where protoporphyrin is converted to haem by ferrochelatase, deficiency of which leads to a high accumulation of protoporphyrin which is highly photosensitizing. Red blood cells (RBC) and faeces show increased levels of protoporphyrins. Fresh RBCs fluoresce coral red when examined in a dark room under ultraviolet light.

Approximately 10 per cent of patients with EPP may have underlying haemolytic anaemia, hypersplenism and cholelithiasis (including in young children). Associated liver disease is common, but fortunately rarely leads to fatal hepatic failure requiring hepatic transplantation.

Management includes education concerning photoprotective measures to prevent exposure to ultraviolet and visible light. Patients should avoid any unnecessary exposure to sunlight and should wear photoprotective clothing / wide-brimmed hat. If possible, tinted windows should be installed.

Patients / medical practitioners should remember that other strong sources of light can also trigger symptoms, including indoor fluorescent and halogen lights. Patients with EPP should have strict photoprotection of their skin during surgical procedures, as operating lights can trigger severe attacks. Oral β-carotene can be effective in some patients in reducing photosensitivity.

 KEY POINTS

- EPP is a rare, hereditary autosomal dominant disorder of porphyrin metabolism.
- Patients usually present in childhood with photosensitivity.
- The mainstay of management is photoprotection.

History

A 38-year-old woman presented with a lump in her breast and was diagnosed with peripheral T-cell non-Hodgkin's lymphoma stage 3A. She underwent six cycles of CHOP-21 chemotherapy; however, a PET (positron emission tomography) scan revealed residual disease in her mediastinal lymph nodes. During a planned admission for a BEAM autologous stem cell transplantation she developed a widespread, mildly pruritic skin eruption. The rash started on her upper body and spread distally over 24 hours. She had received pre-conditioning chemotherapy and prophylactic antimicrobials (azithromycin, penicillin, fluconazole, aciclovir) 4 days prior to the onset of the eruption.

Examination

There are multiple erythematous macules and papules scattered diffusely over her trunk and limbs (Fig. 19.1), with relative sparing of her face. There are no pustules, blisters or scaling. The eruption blanches on pressure.

INVESTIGATIONS

		Normal
White cell count	6.68×10^9/L	$4.0–11.0 \times 10^9$/L
Haemoglobin	10.7 g/dL	11.5–16.5 g/dL
Platelets	141×10^9/L	$150–450 \times 10^9$/L
Neutrophils	4.92×10^9/L	$2.2–6.3 \times 10^9$/L
Lymphocytes	0.22×10^9/L	$1.3–4.0 \times 10^9$/L
Eosinophils	1.49×10^9/L	$0–0.4 \times 10^9$/L
C-reactive protein	42 mg/L	<5 mg/L
Renal and liver function	Normal	
Skin biopsy	A dense perivascular infiltrate of lymphocytes and eosinophils around the upper dermal blood vessels	

Questions

- What is the diagnosis?
- What is the most likely cause of her sudden-onset rash?
- How would you manage this patient?

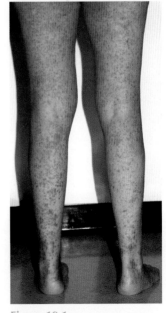

Figure 19.1

The patient has developed a drug rash called toxic erythema; this was confirmed histologically from the skin biopsy. This is the most common type of cutaneous drug eruption. Classically, it spreads in a craniocaudal direction and is mildly pruritic. The rash is symmetrical and consists of a myriad of very small erythematous papules and macules. The individual lesions blanch on pressure. There are no blisters or pustules, the palms and soles are spared. Toxic erythema usually starts within two weeks of taking a new medication. Sudden-onset widespread rashes are usually 'reactive' with the two most common underlying causes being 'drugs or bugs'.

The key to identifying the culprit drug is the taking of a detailed history of the patient's medications and the time course over which each was started in relation to the onset of the rash. In this case the drug responsible is penicillin. If possible, the culprit drug should be stopped; however, if the drug is vital for the patient's underlying condition then toxic erythema can be managed with a moderately potent topical steroid and emollients. Usually the rash fades over a few weeks with desquamation.

KEY POINTS

- Toxic erythema is the most common type of drug rash.
- The rash spreads in a craniocaudal direction and consists of erythematous macules and papules.
- Common culprit drugs include antibiotics, anticonvulsants, allopurinol, non-steroidal anti-inflammatories, and thiazides.

History

A 40-year-old woman is referred to the dermatology clinic with a history of erythematous skin lesions appearing on her face, neck and chest over the past six weeks. She complains of a burning and slight itching with the onset of new lesions that then settle over a few weeks leaving marked pigmentation on her skin. Intermittently she has developed new lesions in addition to the old lesions flaring. She had no previous history of skin problems. Past medical history includes mild asthma, hayfever and hypertension. Her medication includes becotide and salbutamol inhalers, simvastatin, atenolol and ramipril; the latter was commenced within the last 2 months to help control her hypertension.

Examination

There are multiple annular hyperpigmented macular lesions on the skin over her face, neck and upper chest (Fig. 20.1). No new erythematous lesions or recently 'reactivated' lesions are apparent at the time of this clinic appointment.

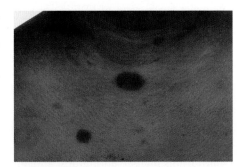

Figure 20.1

🔍 INVESTIGATIONS

Histology from her skin biopsy showed a resolving inflammatory interface dermatitis (at the junction between the epidermis and the dermis) with numerous lymphocytes and dying keratinocytes (civatte bodies). There was scattered melanin pigment in the upper dermis.

Questions

- What is the diagnosis?
- What is the likely cause?
- How would you manage this patient?

This patient was diagnosed with a fixed drug eruption (FDE), which is an interesting phenomenon where exposure to a particular medication leads to annular erythematous skin lesion(s) which heal with pigmentation. Repeated exposure to the drug invariably causes reactivation of the old skin lesion(s) and may cause new ones to appear. Solitary skin lesions most commonly occur in FDE and preferentially occur on the genitalia and lips. This patient had the multiple FDE variant where lesions more frequently appear on the arms and trunk. There are reports of FDE lesions occurring on the genitals in patients who are allergic to their sexual partner's medication.

The morphology of the skin lesions in FDE is somewhat variable, however. Classically they are circular or oval, macular or bullous and heal with pigmentation. Some FDE eruptions can be so inflammatory that central skin necrosis can result.

The exact mechanism of FDE is not known. Our current understanding is that the medication acts as a hapten which binds to keratinocytes within the epidermis. This triggers the release of pro-inflammatory cytokines which attract T-cells (CD4 and CD8) into the affected skin site. Reactivation of the skin lesions in response to re-exposure to the medication activates memory T-cells at the identical skin site(s). Histological appearances of involved skin show the action is at the dermoepidermal junction.

The onset of FDE usually starts within two weeks of commencing a new medication. In this case the most likely culprit is the ramipril owing to the temporal relationship between commencement of the drug and the onset of the skin lesions. The most common culprit drugs include antibiotics, anticonvulsants and analgesics. However, FDE has been reported as being associated with many other preparations including over-the-counter medications, supplements, minerals and even foods.

The diagnosis of FDE is usually straightforward with a good history and classic clinical signs. If it is unclear which medication may be the culprit then an oral challenge can be useful. Histological appearances from lesional skin can help support the clinical diagnosis of FDE but is usually not diagnostic. Once the culprit medication has been identified this should be stopped. A potent topical steroid can be applied to any active lesions, which will help settle any symptoms and inflammation rapidly.

 KEY POINTS

- FDE lesions on the skin are reactivated each time the culprit drug is ingested.
- Lesions are frequently solitary and have a predilection for the lips and genitals.
- Skin lesions are often annular with central blistering/necrosis that settles with pigmentation.

History

A 39-year-old man is referred by his GP to the on-call dermatologist with a 3-day history of a sore throat, painful mouth and blistering rash. One week prior to the onset of his painful mouth and rash he developed a sore on his upper lip. The sore on his upper lip and widespread blistering eruption had first occurred at the age of 7 years and had erupted on four previous occasions. He feels well in himself but is having difficulty eating due to his painful mouth. His past medical history includes diet-controlled diabetes, hypertension and hypercholesterolaemia. He was commenced on amlodipine and simvastatin two years previously.

Examination

Annular target-like lesions are seen over his lips (Fig. 21.1) and blistering annular lesions over his hands, elbows and trunk (Fig. 21.2). Within his mouth are painful blisters (Fig. 21.3) and eroded erythematous ulcers.

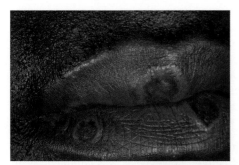

Figure 21.1

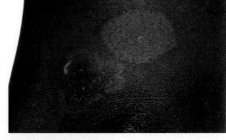

Figure 21.2

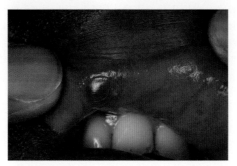

Figure 21.3

🔍 INVESTIGATIONS

He is apyrexial, blood pressure is 140/88 mmHg, and pulse is normal. Viral and bacterial swabs, and skin biopsy were taken through a blister.

Questions

- What is the underlying diagnosis and what secondary phenomenon has occurred?
- How would you treat the patient initially?
- What management would you instigate to prevent further similar attacks?

When patients present with a sore ulcerated mouth the differential diagnoses include aphthous ulcers, viral stomatitis such as caused by herpes simplex virus (HSV), shingles (herpes zoster virus), Behçet's disease, immunobullous disease (pemphigus vulgaris), vitamin/iron deficiency, neutropenia, and adverse drug reactions.

The clue to the underlying cause of this patient's oral ulceration was the preceding sore on his upper lip – herpes labialis ('cold sore') caused by HSV type 1 was isolated from a viral swab. Subsequent to his HSV infection he developed erythema multiforme (EM). This manifested in this patient as oral ulceration and target lesions on his lips and focal skin sites. Histology of the skin biopsy showed marked dermal oedema and subepidermal blisters containing neutrophils and eosinophils.

Target lesions of EM are typically seen on the face, elbows, knees, palms and soles (so-called 'acral sites'). The lesions themselves consist of erythematous annular rings with a central papule or vesicle. However, as the name suggests, the cutaneous eruption can be variable in appearance (multiforme).

With EM there may or may not be involvement of mucous membranes. EM minor is cutaneous involvement at the typical acral sites; EM major has the same cutaneous eruption ($<$10 per cent epidermal detachment) plus involvement of one or more mucous membrane sites. This can be distinguished from Stevens–Johnson syndrome that has 10–30 per cent skin surface area with epidermal detachment and always significant mucous membrane involvement. Drugs rather than infections are more commonly associated with the onset of Stevens–Johnson syndrome. The cause of EM is usually an infection rather than a medication, with HSV and *Mycoplasma pneumoniae* most commonly implicated.

This patient presented too late to be treated with aciclovir for his herpes labialis (which should be initiated in the first 72 hours to be effective), however he was commenced on aciclovir 400 mg daily as secondary prophylaxis against further episodes. Moderately potent topical steroid was applied to all the EM lesions and he rinsed his mouth with the NSAID benzydiamine hydrochloride (Difflam) mouthwash, four times daily. Some patients develop recurrent EM despite prophylactic aciclovir. In these cases a systemic immunosuppressive agent such as azathioprine or ciclosporin may be needed to prevent further attacks of EM.

 KEY POINTS

- Erythema multiforme (EM) is a reactive skin eruption that is usually the result of an underlying infection.
- Although the appearance of the skin lesions can be variable, target-like lesions at acral sites are classically seen.
- EM with mucous membrane involvement (lips, genitals, nose) is termed EM major.

History

A 35-year-old female presents with a 2-day history of a sore throat, malaise and a rash. The cutaneous eruption has spread rapidly over the two days to involve her trunk, limbs and face. Her eyes feel gritty and sore. Her lips have become crusted and painful. Three weeks previously her antiepileptic medication had been changed from topiramate to carbamazepine.

Examination

The cutaneous eruption consists of dusky erythema which is patchy on her face and limbs but more confluent over her trunk. Between 20 and 30 per cent of the skin surface is involved in the eruption. Blisters are seen centrally within erythematous, atypical, target-like lesions and there are purpuric macules. Nikolsky's sign is positive (sloughing-off of the epidermis under lateral pressure). She has chelitis with erythema, crusting and bleeding. There are erosions and small areas of skin necrosis (Fig. 22.1). The nasal mucosa and genital tract are spared.

INVESTIGATIONS

Her temperature is 38.4 °C, blood pressure 138/80 mmHg, and pulse 96 bpm. A skin biopsy was taken for histology and immunofluorescence. She has mildly deranged liver function.

		Normal
C-reactive protein	43 mg/L	<5.0 mg/L
Erythrocyte sedimentation rate	112 mm/h	1–10 mm/h
Haemoglobin	10.6 g/dL	11.5–16.5 g/dL
Platelets	330 × 10⁹/L	150–450 × 10⁹/L
Ferritin	577 µg/L	20–200 µg/L

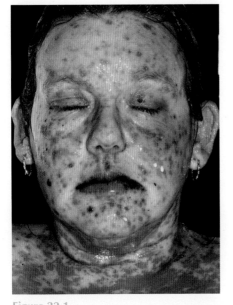

Figure 22.1

Questions

- What is the most likely cause of this rapid-onset skin eruption?
- What management plan would you instigate?
- Which healthcare professionals should ideally be involved in her care?

This patient has developed Stevens–Johnson syndrome (SJS) secondary to carbamazepine. SJS is a severe, immune-complex mediated, drug hypersensitivity eruption that affects the skin and mucous membranes. Patients feel unwell and should be admitted to hospital for high-dependency care. SJS usually develops within two months of commencing a new medication. Patients characteristically develop a sore throat, eyes, lips and genitals as the mucosae become inflamed and eroded. Skin lesions affect 10–30 per cent of the skin surface with a variable morphology: erythematous macules, atypical target lesions with central blisters, dusky purpuric lesions, erosions and necrosis. As the skin becomes denuded there is a high risk of secondary bacterial infection.

Patients with SJS need management in hospital by a multidisciplinary team including dermatologists, high-dependency doctors and nurses, ophthalmologists and oral physicians. This patient also required care from the neurologists to determine and monitor an alternative anti-epileptic medication.

The management of SJS is essentially supportive. The culprit medication should be stopped immediately (if the culprit is unclear then all mediations should be stopped if possible). Patients require intensive nursing care with hourly applications of topical 50:50 white soft paraffin with liquid paraffin, non-adherent dressings to denuded areas and a non-adherent bodysuit to help reduce cutaneous pain and secondary infection. Patients should be kept in a warm room and fluid balance monitored. Chlorhexidine mouthwash, regular eye drops, and supportive nutrition may be required. Active treatments may include prednisolone, methyl-prednisolone, intravenous immunoglobulin and/or ciclosporin.

 KEY POINTS

- SJS is a serious drug hypersensitivity reaction that requires high-dependency care.
- Skin lesions are of variable appearance but develop rapidly with mucous membrane involvement.
- Management is supportive plus treatment with oral prednisolone or other immunosuppressants.

History

A 34-year-old woman who was 24 weeks pregnant developed sudden-onset sore eyes, mouth and genitalia associated with blisters on her skin. She was admitted to hospital by the obstetricians who referred her to the on-call dermatologist. The patient was diagnosed with HIV at antenatal screening and had been commenced on HAART (highly active antiretroviral therapy) – Combivir and nevirapine – 2 weeks ago. Over the last 24 hours she has felt unwell with a fever, malaise, sore throat, gritty eyes and a painful stomatitis. Initially she had a few blisters on her face and upper trunk but over a few hours these spread to involve extensive areas of her trunk and limbs.

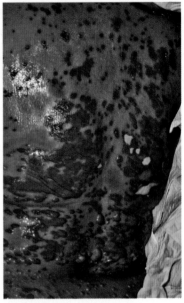

Figure 23.1

Examination

She is unwell and distressed. Her temperature is 38.2 °C, blood pressure 180/100 mmHg and pulse rate 110 beats/min. There is crusting and bleeding of her lips, her conjunctiva are severely injected and she has inflamed nasal mucosa. The genital region is inflamed and erythematous. She has numerous flaccid and tense blisters over her face, limbs and trunk with many areas becoming confluent with small areas of complete tissue necrosis and skin loss (Fig. 23.1). More than 30 per cent of her skin surface is affected, Nikolsky's sign is positive.

INVESTIGATIONS		
		Normal
White cell count	11.15 × 10⁹/L	4.00–11.0 × 10⁹/L
Haemoglobin	9.7 g/dL	11.5–16.5 g/dL
Platelets	211 × 10⁹/L	150–450 × 10⁹/L
Neutrophils	8.29 × 10⁹/L	2.20–6.30 × 10⁹/L
Lymphocytes	1.28 × 10⁹/L	1.30–4.00 × 10⁹/L
Eosinophils	0.88 × 10⁹/L	0–0.4 × 10⁹/L
C-reactive protein	147 mg/L	<5 mg/L
HIV viral load	79 869 copies/mL	
CD4 lymphocyte count	229	

A cardiotocography (CTG) examination was normal.

Urea, bicarbonate and glucose tests were all normal.

A skin biopsy was taken.

Questions

- What is the most likely cause of this patient's sudden-onset skin eruption?
- What is the prognosis for the patient and her baby?
- How would you manage them?

This presentation with widespread skin loss is typical of drug-induced toxic epidermal necrolysis (TEN). Nikolsky's sign is positive when lateral pressure is applied to the skin and the top layer sloughs off, and is found in TEN, Stevens–Johnson syndrome and staphylococcal scalded skin syndrome and immuno-bullous diseases. The most likely culprit drug here is the antiretroviral nevarapine. Currently physicians are unable to predict which patients will develop severe drug eruptions; however, they are more common in patients with HIV. The trigger antigen sets off a cascade of cell-mediated immune reactions including the activation of cytotoxic lymphocytes and natural killer cells resulting in full-thickness skin necrosis (confirmed on the skin biopsy).

TEN is a dermatological emergency. Patients should be managed in the intensive care unit by a multidisciplinary team including a dermatologist. Many patients with TEN require sedation and ventilation. The offending drug should be stopped immediately. Topical 50:50 white soft paraffin with liquid paraffin should be applied hourly to all the skin, topical antibiotics and non-adherent dressings (Jelonet®) should be applied to denuded areas. Patients should be kept in a warm room. Fluid and enteral nutrition are essential to compensate for high insensible fluid losses and high protein demands. The evidence for other proactive interventions are mainly anecdotal: many units will treat patients with a total of 2–4 mg/kg of intravenous immunoglobulin over 4 days and 3 mg/kg per day of ciclosporin.

TEN has a reported mortality rate of around 20–40 per cent. The mortality rate for any individual patient can be estimated by calculating their SCORTEN – based on seven criteria: > 40 years of age, pulse > 120 bpm, underlying malignancy, > 10 per cent body surface involved, urea > 10 mmol/L, bicarbonate < 20 mmol/L and glucose > 14 mmol/L. The higher the number of these criteria the patient has, the worse the prognosis (mortality: 1/7 = 3 per cent, 2/7 = 12 per cent, 3/7 = 35 per cent, 4/7 = 58 per cent, 5–7/7 = 90 per cent).

This patient had a normal healthy baby delivered at term by caesarean section and was switched to Kaletra, lamivudine and tenofovir.

 KEY POINTS

- TEN is a dermatological emergency requiring meticulous skin care and supportive therapy.
- Patients usually require sedation and ventilation on the intensive care unit.
- The patient's prognosis can be estimated by calculating their SCORTEN.

History

A 28-year-old female was admitted to hospital with viral encephalitis. During her illness she developed a saggital sinus thrombosis and resultant epilepsy. She was commenced on anticoagulants and phenytoin. Six weeks after her hospital admission she develops an itchy and painful rash on her face, trunk and limbs. At the time of referral to the dermatology team she has an ongoing fever, headache and general malaise. She has no previous medical history of note.

Examination

The patient's face and ears are erythematous with marked oedema; elsewhere she has a widespread maculopapular eruption (Fig. 24.1). There is lymphadenopathy in the cervical, axillary and inguinal regions. Mucous membranes are normal and no blisters are seen. Her temperature is 39.1 °C.

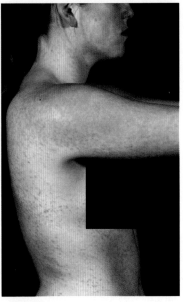

Figure 24.1

INVESTIGATIONS

		Normal
White cell count	30.66 × 10⁹/L	4.0–11.0 × 10⁹/L
Haemoglobin	11.7 g/dL	11.5–16.5 g/dL
Platelets	485 × 10⁹/L	150–450 × 10⁹/L
Neutrophils	23.40 × 10⁹/L	2.20–6.30 × 10⁹/L
Lymphocytes	2.09 × 10⁹/L	1.3–4.0 × 10⁹/L
Eosinophils	3.29 × 10⁹/L	0.00–0.40 × 10⁹/L
C-reactive protein	13.8 mg/L	< 5 mg/L
Erythrocyte sedimentation rate	3.0 mm/h	1–10 mm/h
Albumin	38 g/L	35–50 g/L
Alkaline phosphatase	196 IU/L	30–130 IU/L
Aspartate transaminase	144 IU/L	10–50 IU/L
γ-glutamyl transferase	876 IU/L	1–55 IU/L
INR (international normalized ratio)	2.44	0.90–1.20

A skin biopsy was taken.

Questions

- What is the dermatological diagnosis?
- What management would you initiate?

This patient was diagnosed with a drug hypersensitivity syndrome called DRESS (drug rash with eosinophilia and systemic symptoms). The symptoms and signs of DRESS may be misdiagnosed as an ongoing infection as patients having a swinging temperature, malaise, lymphadenopathy, a skin rash and eosinophilia. The systemic part of the syndrome can manifest with internal organ involvement most commonly liver, lung or kidneys. The mortality rate is around 10 per cent.

The cutaneous manifestations of DRESS can vary quite widely. However, most patients have quite erythematous and oedematous skin especially in the head and neck region. Patients may present with marked oedema around their eyes and ears. The morphology of the widespread skin eruption may be macular, papular, coalescing plaques, occasionally vesicular or pustular lesions, and there may be areas of desquamation. Mucous membranes are spared. The rash may be mildly itchy, the skin may feel tight and uncomfortable.

Marked reactive lymphadenopathy is usually present in the cervical and axillary lymph node basins. The patient's fever is usually marked and swinging. Patients look and feel unwell. Eosinophilia and raised liver function tests are commonly seen but may lag behind the onset of the skin eruption.

The most common drugs implicated in DRESS include antibiotics and anticonvulsants. DRESS usually occurs within 8–12 weeks after commencing the culprit drug. The phenytoin was the drug implicated in this case and was therefore stopped immediately. The patient was treated with pulsed intravenous methyl prednisolone (1 g daily for 3 days) and then a tapering course of oral prednisolone starting at 40 mg daily and reducing down slowly over 6 weeks.

There is rapid normalization of the patient's temperature and eosinophil count with commencement of systemic steroids. The hepatitis may not settle for several weeks, and may even deteriorate further before settling. In severe cases of reactive hepatitis in DRESS patients may eventually require liver transplantation due to the acute liver damage.

 KEY POINTS

- DRESS can often present with clinical signs and symptoms that may be misdiagnosed as an infection.
- A lag of 8–12 weeks occurs between starting the culprit medication and the onset of DRESS.
- DRESS has a 10 per cent mortality rate; the culprit drug should be stopped immediately and systemic steroids given.

CASE 25: ACUTE-ONSET MULTIPLE PUSTULES ON A BACKGROUND OF ERYTHEMATOUS SKIN

History

A 41-year-old woman presents to the on-call medical team with a fever and mild malaise. She complains of a sore rash with pustules appearing on her trunk and limbs over the past 24 hours. She was previously fit and well with no history of previous skin problems. There is no family history of note. She had been taking a herbal preparation over the past few months but this had stopped 3 weeks ago. She is currently taking a course of penicillin prescribed by her GP 3 days earlier.

Examination

The patient has a temperature and looks unwell. She has a widespread erythema over her trunk and limbs that is studded with multiple, small monomorphic pustules (Fig. 25.1). There is a predilection for the flexural areas. Nikolsky's sign is negative. Mucous membranes, nails and scalp are normal. Her temperature is 38.4 °C.

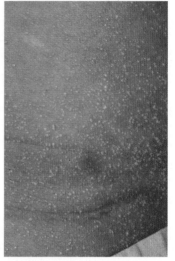

Figure 25.1

INVESTIGATIONS

		Normal
White cell count	16.61 × 10⁹/L	4.00–11.0 × 10⁹/L
Haemoglobin	10.2 g/dL	11.5–16.5 g/dL
Platelets	692 × 10⁹/L	150–450 × 10⁹/L
Neutrophils	15.26 × 10⁹/L	2.20–6.30 × 10⁹/L
Lymphocytes	0.85 × 10⁹/L	1.30–4.00 × 10⁹/L
Erythrocyte sedimentation rate	22 mm/h	1–10 mm/h
C-reactive protein	32 mg/L	<5 mg/L
Skin swabs and skin biopsy were taken.		

Questions

- What is the cutaneous diagnosis?
- What is the likely cause?
- How would you manage this patient?

This patient presented with a very dramatic tender skin eruption called AGEP (acute generalized exanthematous pustulosis). This is a pustular drug eruption, most likely caused in this case by penicillin. AGEP is characterized by multiple pin-point pustules which are very monomorphic in nature and appear in sheets on an erythematous background. There is often accentuation in the flexural areas such as axillae and groin. Swabs are negative for organisms as the pustules are sterile. In contrast infected cutaneous pustules tend to be at different stages of evolution varying in size and shape, the erythema tends to be localized around each pustule rather than diffuse; lesions may be crusted.

The differential diagnosis includes acute pustular psoriasis. Some patients may have a past history of psoriasis (usually the chronic plaque form) in which the skin suddenly becomes unstable (this can be triggered by oral prednisolone) and develops multiple sterile pustules within the psoriatic plaques. Pustules are usually prominent around the periphery of the areas of erythema rather than as sheets of pustules throughout. Rarely, it may be difficult to differentiate between AGEP and pustular psoriasis, as some patients' first presentation of psoriasis may be with the acute pustular form.

Pateints with AGEP frequently have a fever and mild to moderate malaise. Blood tests usually show a neutrophilia and a mildly raised CRP. Patients may therefore be misdiagnosed as having a skin infection due to staphylococcal bacteria. Histology from the skin biopsy shows subcorneal collections of neutrophils, which is supportive of the diagnosis of AGEP. In psoriasis there is usually an associated thickening of the epidermal skin layer – so-called acanthosis – which is absent in AGEP.

The drug implicated in AGEP should be stopped immediately if at all possible. Pustules usually resolve over 1–2 weeks. To speed the cutaneous recovery, systemic corticosteroids should be given. Topical treatment with 50:50 white soft paraffin with liquid paraffin should be applied to the skin every 2 hours in the acute phase. Secondary infection by *Staphylococcus* bacteria to eroded areas can occur before the skin heals. In the meantime patients can loose heat and fluids through their impaired skin barrier causing high insensible fluid losses.

 KEY POINTS

- AGEP is an acute-onset drug eruption characterized by sheets of monomorphic pustules on red skin.
- The pustules in AGEP are sterile and represent a toxic drug reaction and not a skin infection.
- The culprit drug should be stopped and systemic/topical steroids used to treat the patient.

CASE 26: ACUTE NON-BLANCHING CUTANEOUS ERUPTION ASSOCIATED WITH A SORE THROAT

History

A 62-year-old man presents to the accident and emergency department with a 2-day history of an asymptomatic skin eruption appearing mainly on his trunk and limbs. It seems to have started after visiting his local swimming pool and he had wondered if the chlorine in the water may have triggered the skin rash. He is otherwise fit and well but has recently had a sore throat and temperature but no cough. He has no previous history of skin problems. He is referred to the on-call dermatology team.

Examination

There is a widespread eruption mainly on the lower limbs and trunk but also to a lesser extent on his arms. The morphology of the rash is purple and non-blanching; lesions are starting to coalesce and are mainly macular but some are papular (Fig. 26.1). His tonsils are erythematous with some surface exudate and he has tender cervical lymphadenopathy. His temperature is 38.7 °C.

🔍 INVESTIGATIONS

Throat swab, urine dipstick and skin biopsy were taken.

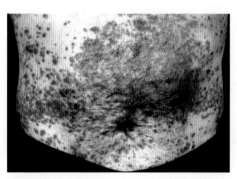

Figure 26.1

Questions

- What is the likely cause of the skin eruption?
- What pathological process would be seen on the skin histopathology?
- What is the differential diagnosis of this skin rash?

Non-blanching skin eruptions usually indicate bleeding into the skin, blockage of cutaneous blood vessels or reduced blood flow (viscosity/stasis). The underlying cause may be benign such as pressure on the skin, or serious such as bacterial meningitis.

Small pin-point areas of bleeding into the skin, so-called 'petechiae', can occur due to leakage from small cutaneous capillaries (capillaritis), pressure on the skin (from tight bandages/compression stockings) or vascular damage due to infections. Larger areas of bleeding into the skin (ecchymoses) can occur on the limbs of elderly patients following minor trauma, as their skin is thin and fragile.

Macular areas of purple non-blanching skin are usually the result of red cell leakage or bleeding (low platelet count). Palpable purpura by contrast is usually associated with an acute inflammatory process such as vasculitis. Acute and severe vascular damage may result in skin necrosis.

This patient had acute vasculitis (leucocytoclastic vasculitis), which is inflammation of the blood vessels. This inflammation leads to leakage of red cells and ultimately blockage of skin blood vessels. Skin biopsy is extremely helpful in confirming the clinical suspicion of vasculitis. Histology from affected skin shows tissue swelling, perivascular inflammation and fibrin blocking cutaneous blood vessels. Neutrophils around the vessels are frequently killed (leucocytoclasis) and remnants of them ('nuclear dust') are seen scattered in the dermis.

The throat swab from this patient confirmed a streptococcal infection, which is the likely underlying cause of his vasculitis. He was treated with oral penicillin V and potent topical steroids.

The differential diagnosis of a vasculitic rash includes bacterial meningitis, *Streptococcus*, hepatitis C/B, autoimmune diseases (lupus, polyarteritis nodosa, rheumatoid), drug reaction and malignancy.

Investigations of cutaneous vasculitis might include the following: skin biopsy, urine dipstick (for blood/casts), full blood count, erythrocyte sedimentation rate, renal/liver function, streptococcal serology (ASOT), hepatitis serology, antinuclear antibodies (ANA), extractable nuclear antibodies (ENA), antineutrophil cytoplasmic antibodies (ANCA), rheumatoid factor, coagulation screen, antiphospholipid antibodies, blood pressure, and chest X-ray.

 KEY POINTS

- Acute-onset non-blanching purple skin eruptions can indicate a serious underlying cause.
- Skin biopsy can help to distinguish between true vasculitis and simple blood vessel leakage.
- A vasculitis screen may help to elucidate the underlying cause.

History

A 47-year-old woman is seen in the dermatology clinic with a 5-month history of itchy eruption consisting of lesions mainly on her feet but also scattered on her legs. The rest of her skin is unaffected. She does not complain of any symptoms in her mouth or involving the genital area. On direct questioning she had noticed that some of her nails have become slightly brittle and are liable to splitting. No one else in the family is currently affected, although she thinks her mother had suffered with a similar skin eruption some years previously. She is otherwise well and not taking any regular medication.

Examination

There are multiple, discrete, purplish, shiny flat-topped papules over the dorsum of her feet; some of the lesions have a lacy white pattern over their surface (Fig. 27.1). Further similar lesions are seen scattered on her lower legs; some of the papules are clustered in a linear fashion demonstrating Koebner's phenomenon. A number of her fingernails have longitudinal ridges on them with 'V-shaped' nicks. Her mouth, genital region and scalp are all normal.

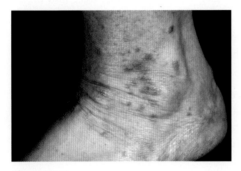

Figure 27.1

Questions
- What is the diagnosis?
- What triggers are known to be associated with this skin disease?
- What are the treatment options for this patient?

This woman was diagnosed with cutaneous lichen planus. The aetiology of the eruption is unknown; however, it is thought to be an immunologically mediated disease and is known to be associated with autoimmune diseases and hepatitis C. Recent articles suggest that 16 per cent of patients with lichen planus have underlying hepatitis C. In addition numerous medications have been implicated in triggering lichenoid drug reactions including diuretics, β-blockers, NSAIDs, angiotensin converting enzyme inhibitors, statins and tetracyclines. A familial tendency has been reported in association with certain human leucocyte (HLA) types being implicated including HLA-B7, HLA-DR1/10.

Clinically lichen planus presents with an insidious onset, mildly to intensely pruritic eruptions especially seen on the flexor aspects of the wrists but also scattered on the limbs and trunk. The lesions themselves are usually papules that are purplish in colour, shiny and firm on palpation. There may be a fine white lacy pattern of scale on the surface of the lesions (Wickham's striae). Lesions may form discrete nodules/plaques and become quite hyperkeratotic. A scarring alopecia can develop due to scalp involvement, so-called lichen planopilaris. In addition to the cutaneous eruption, patients may have involvement of the mouth and genital mucosae with sore erosions and ulceration. Nails changes may also feature and are characterized by longitudinal ridges and brittle 'V-shaped' nicks in the distal nail plate.

The diagnosis is usually made on clinical grounds. However, histological features seen on a skin biopsy can be helpful in distinguishing between lichen planus and lichenoid drug eruptions when a drug trigger is suspected.

Most lichen planus settles within months to years and responds well to potent topical steroids, phototherapy or short courses of oral prednisolone. Orogenital involvement, however, may be more persistent and recalcitrant and may require prolonged systemic immunosuppressant therapy such as mycophenolate mofetil.

 KEY POINTS

- Lichen planus is an itchy papular eruption of insidious onset.
- In extensive or atypical disease think about a possible drug trigger or underlying hepatitis C.
- Cutaneous lesions respond to potent topical steroids but orogenital disease is more recalcitrant.

History

A 67-year-old woman presents to the accident and emergency department with a 6-day history of severe, painful and progressive blistering. She had attended her GP eight weeks earlier with a worsening 'burning itchy' eruption. She had been diagnosed with urticaria and been started on a regular antihistamine with no benefit. Two weeks ago she had attended her dental practitioner with painful oral erosions, and is awaiting specialist review.

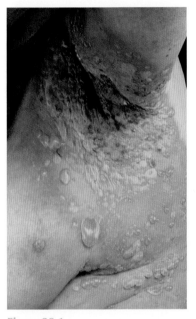

Her past medical history includes a cholecystectomy and borderline abnormal thyroid function tests, for which she is on no therapy currently. She is an ex-smoker. There are no other remarkable features in her history.

Examination

The patient is clearly uncomfortable at rest and it is painful for her to move during the examination. She has two small (< 5 mm) healing erosions on her right buccal mucosa and a fresh tense blister (~7 mm) on her hard palate. The rest of her oral examination is normal. She has a symmetrical erythematous urticated eruption over the lateral aspects of her trunk, her submammary area, medial upper arms, and thighs and central back. Within these erythematous lesions there are multiple tense fluid-filled vesicles (< 5 mm) and bullae (> 5 mm) (Fig. 28.1). Her genital mucosa is normal. The remainder of her physical examination is normal.

Figure 28.1

INVESTIGATIONS		
		Normal
Haemoglobin	15.6 g/dL	13.3–17.7 g/dL
Mean corpuscular volume	93 fL	90–99 fL
White cell count	13.4×10^9/L	$3.9–10.6 \times 10^9$/L
Platelets	512×10^9/L	$150–440 \times 10^9$/L
Differential white cell count	Eosinophils 9%	1–3%
Blood film:	Eosinophilic leucocytosis	
Urea and electrolytes	Normal	
Liver function tests	Normal	

Questions

- In addition to establishing a diagnosis, what are the immediate priorities in the management of this patient?
- What are the likely diagnosis and the possible differential diagnoses?
- What is the long-term prognosis?

This is clearly a widespread, evolving and aggressive, blistering eruption. In addition to establishing a diagnosis and ruling out any underlying medical disorders, the priorities for this patient are pain relief and prevention of infection. Pain relief would include simple measures such as reducing friction to eroded areas of the skin (with easy-release dressings and/or greasy emollients) and minimizing activity, as well as pharmacological pain relief. Preventing infection can be challenging: barrier nursing and use of topical antiseptics such as potassium permanganate, triclosan and chlorhexidine, particularly when washing, are frequently advocated.

The age of the patient, her history and presentation, and eosinophilia are highly suggestive of a diagnosis of bullous pemphigoid. Other autoimmune bullous diseases could be considered in the differential diagnosis, in particular: inflammatory epidermolysis bullosa acquisita (a mucous membrane pemphigoid, which often has a more insidious onset with more mucosal involvement than skin); erythema multiforme major (usually more haemorrhagic mucosal involvement and targetoid lesions); and bullous vasculitis (usually purpuric skin lesions in association with blistering, especially of the lower extremities). Occasionally bullous pemphigoid can be associated with underlying conditions such as inflammatory bowel disease or occult malignancy or be provoked by medication (e.g. furosemide, ACE inhibitors, and recently anti-TNF monoclonal antibody therapy).

Bullous pemphigoid is characterized by circulating and tissue-bound pathogenic anti-cutaneous basement membrane zone antibodies. These can be detected by immunofluorescence studies (on skin and serum). Figure 28.2 demonstrates positive green fluorescence of tissue-bound antibodies along the cutaneous basement membrane. Immunosuppression with systemic corticosteroids and steroid-sparing agents is the cornerstone of treatment; although for patients with milder or more localized disease superpotent topical corticosteroids alone may be sufficient to achieve disease control. Remission over a period of years is expected; however, prognosis is adversely affected in the elderly by their frequent co-morbidities.

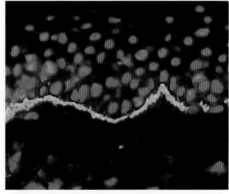

Figure 28.2

Further investigations to confirm the diagnosis of bullous pemphigoid

Test	Tissue	Result in bullous pemphigoid
Histopathology	Lesional skin	Subepidermal blister with eosinophil-rich inflammatory infiltrate
Direct immunofluorescence	Peri-lesional skin	IgG and complement C3 deposition in a linear band at the dermal–epidermal junction
Indirect immunofluorescence	Serum	Presence of IgG circulating targeting the skin basement membrane component

KEY POINTS

- Bullous pemphigoid frequently affects elderly individuals, presenting as painful tense bullae on a pruritic urticated base. Mucosal involvement is not usually a major feature.
- As well as the necessary investigations to confirm the diagnosis, co-morbidities and occult underlying diseases should be sought prior to initiation of immunosuppressive therapy.
- The natural history is for bullous pemphigoid to remit over years, but the adverse effects of immunosuppressive treatment on the elderly can be significant.

History

A 29-year-old lawyer attends the accident and emergency department with a sudden and severe skin eruption. She has a 3-day history of a rapidly progressing, painful, erosive eruption affecting her upper trunk and intertriginous (groin and axillae) areas. She is unable to sleep and finds dressing and undressing difficult as her skin 'sticks' to her clothes and then tears off. The eruption is occurring on the background of a 4-month history of painful 'ulcers' in her mouth and on closer questioning also her genital skin, which she had attributed to stress. She has been avoiding hot, spicy or hard food for a couple of months.

She is otherwise well and is on no medication. Her mother has type 2 diabetes and hypertension. Otherwise there is no family history of significant skin or medical disorders.

Examination

She has a widespread skin eruption over her trunk, within her axillae and groin, and involving the inner lips of her vulva. There are multiple discrete and coalescing lesions. The individual lesions are erythematous and tender with overlying erosions, flaccid bullae and friable scale (Fig. 29.1). There are similar erosions involving the mouth, particularly the lips and buccal mucosae. Nikolsky's sign is positive. The remainder of her physical examination is normal.

INVESTIGATIONS		
		Normal
Haemoglobin	12.7 g/dL	13.3–17.7 g/dL
White cell count	16.9 × 10⁹/L	3.9–10.6 × 10⁹/L
Platelets	456 × 10⁹/L	150–440 × 10⁹/L
Blood film:	Lymphocytic leucocytosis	
Erythrocyte sedimentation rate	35 mm/h	<10 mm/h
C-reactive protein	13 mg/L	<5 mg/L
Urinalysis	Trace of blood, protein and leucocytes	

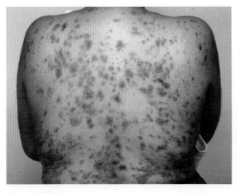

Figure 29.1

Questions

- What is Nikolsky's sign?
- What is the likely diagnosis?
- How would you confirm the diagnosis?
- What is the management?

Nikolsky's sign occurs in patients with active blistering diseases – firm sliding pressure with a finger separates normal-looking epidermis, producing an erosion.

The presence of flaccid blisters on an inflammatory base affecting the skin and mucosa in this age group is most suggestive of a diagnosis of pemphigus vulgaris. Differential diagnoses to consider include other immunobullous diseases such as bullous pemphigoid, linear immunoglobulin A (IgA) disease or dermatitis herpetiformis, erythema multiforme or Stevens–Johnson syndrome. If the lesions were confined to the skin only, pemphigus foliaceous or staphylococcal scalded skin syndrome could be considered.

The diagnosis of pemphigus vulgaris, an intra-epidermal antibody-mediated autoimmune blistering disease, is made on skin biopsy. Histology of a blister shows separation at the suprabasal layer of the epidermis with acantholysis or individual separation of single keratinocytes. Immunofluorescence of peri-lesional skin will demonstrate intercellular IgG throughout the epidermis (Fig. 29.2). Circulating antibodies against desmosomal adhesion molecules (desmogleins 1 and 3) can also be detected, their titre often reflecting the severity of disease.

Pemphigus is a chronic skin disease associated with significant morbidity and formerly, before the synthetic corticosteroid era, a significant mortality due to infection and electrolyte imbalance secondary to fluid loss. Although pemphigus is frequently responsive to systemic steroids, nowadays the side effects of long-term steroid treatment mean that patients are frequently treated with steroid-sparing agents such as azathioprine or mycophenolate mofetil. The use of plasma cell targeting with rituximab, an anti-CD20 monoclonal antibody, has been shown to dramatically reduce circulating autoantibodies and can provide disease control. Extensive skin involvement such as this case may require in-patient management for supportive treatment, skin care, sepsis prevention and pain relief. Specialized dressings which do not adhere to fragile skin may be used, but frequently patients are nursed in such a way as to minimize friction and trauma to the skin.

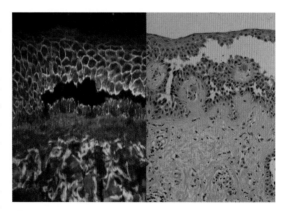

Figure 29.2

> ### KEY POINTS
>
> - Pemphigus vulgaris is a chronic, antibody-mediated autoimmune blistering disease affecting skin and mucosa.
> - Diagnosis is confirmed by the demonstration of bound intercellular antibodies *in vivo* within the epidermis by direct immunofluorescence and circulating antibodies targeting desmogleins 1 and 3 by indirect immunofluorescence.
> - Immunosuppressive treatment particularly aimed at antibody suppression is the cornerstone of therapy. Pain relief and prevention of secondary infection are crucial.

CASE 30: AN ITCHY, VESICULAR EXTENSOR ERUPTION ASSOCIATED WITH MALABSORPTION

History

A 32-year-old carpenter presents with a 3-month history of an itchy, and 'stinging' eruption. He had already been treated with a course of anti-scabies topical therapy and had used a moderately potent topical steroid in combination with antihistamine for 4 weeks with no benefit. He has no significant past medical history and is on no other medication. He comments that the eruption occurs in crops, with small fluid-filled blisters appearing in very itchy patches.

He is one of five siblings, one of his sisters has type 1 diabetes mellitus and his mother is hypothyroid. On systems review he admits to fatigue and 4 kg unintentional weight loss associated with a change in stools over the past several months, which he attributes to stress at work.

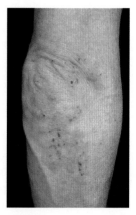

Examination

He has pale, freckled skin, and a symmetrical but patchy eruption, with erythematous and eczematous epidermal change studded with excoriated erosions and crusted papules, clustered particularly over his elbows (Fig. 30.1), buttocks and shoulders. He has no mucosal lesions and no evidence of scabies burrows. The remainder of his physical examination is normal.

Figure 30.1

Questions

- What is this eruption?
- It is a cutaneous manifestation of which gastrointestinal disease?
- What is the management of this patient's condition?

INVESTIGATIONS		
		Normal
Haemoglobin	9.8 g/dL	13.3–17.7 g/dL
Mean corpuscular volume	76 fL	80–99 fL
White cell count	7.3 × 10⁹/L	3.9–10.6 × 10⁹/L
Platelets	566 × 10⁹/L	150–440 × 10⁹/L
Sodium	135 mmol/L	135–145 mmol/L
Potassium	3.8 mmol/L	3.5–5.0 mmol/L
Urea	4.9 mmol/L	2.5–6.7 mmol/L
Creatinine	114 µmol/L	70–120 µmol/L
Albumin	30 g/L	35–50 g/L
Bilirubin	14 mmol/L	3–17 mmol/L
Alanine transaminase	33 IU/L	5–35 IU/L
Alkaline phosphatase	145 IU/L	30–300 IU/L
Thyroid-stimulating hormone	3.1 mIU/L	0.4–4.2 mIU/L
Blood film		Microcytic anaemia and reactive thrombocytosis

The important clues to the diagnosis here are as follows: the distribution of the eruption; the history of pruritic vesicles; the positive family history of probable organ-specific autoimmune disease; his symptoms and blood test results suggestive of an underlying medical disorder. Although the clinical features in Fig. 30.1 are rather non-specific, the lack of response to the treatments already tried in combination with the clues before would all be suggestive of a diagnosis of dermatitis herpetiformis (DH). This is an autoimmune blistering disease characterized by intensely itchy polymorphous vesicular lesions located over the extensor surfaces, back and scalp. It can be difficult to identify vesicles as they are often excoriated, but when the vesicles are present they can be clear, fluid-filled or pus-filled. A routine skin biopsy of peri-lesional skin will show papillary dermal neutrophilic microabcesses. Direct immunofluorescence shows immunoglobulin A (IgA) deposition within the papillary dermis.

DH is a cutaneous manifestation of coeliac disease (gluten-sensitive enteropathy). Both conditions are immunological reactions to ingested gliadin (found in wheat, rye and barley). Serology to detect circulating anti-endomysial and anti-tissue transglutaminase IgA antibodies help to confirm the diagnosis, but a small bowel biopsy should also be performed. Occasionally the features of DH precede the pathological small bowel features of coeliac disease.

A gluten-free diet (GFD) is the treatment of choice for both DH and coeliac disease; importantly it has a protective effect against small bowel lymphoma. Dapsone therapy may be required to gain control of the skin disease. However, after several months of compliance with a GFD this need is usually eliminated.

Autoimmune disorders associated with DH and coeliac disease

- Pernicious anaemia
- Sjögren's syndrome
- Lupus erythematosus
- Thyroiditis
- Diabetes mellitus (type 1)
- Rheumatoid arthritis and juvenile rheumatoid arthritis and juvenile idiopathic arthritis

---

 KEY POINTS

- Dermatitis herpetiformis (DH) is an autoimmune blistering disease and manifestation of gluten sensitive enteropathy.
- DH is associated with a personal or family history of other organ-specific autoimmune diseases.
- The characteristic eruption is composed of intensely pruritic vesicles clustering over extensor surfaces. However, secondary changes due to excoriation may predominate.

History

A 31-year-old woman is referred urgently by her local antenatal service complaining of an 8-day history of extensive and severe itchiness associated with an evolving tender eruption, which began on the palms of her hands and has spread along the inner aspects of her arms and now involves her trunk. She is at 21 weeks' gestation with her second pregnancy.

Her first child is now 2 years old and was born at 38 weeks +3 days by normal vaginal delivery. Her postpartum period, however, was complicated by a similar widespread pruritic eruption, which blistered within her axillae and upper arms. That eruption began 2 days post-delivery and had responded completely to a potent topical steroid within 10 days. She is otherwise well. Her only medication is an iron and folate supplement that was started before conception.

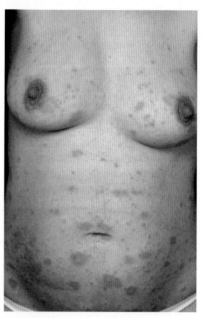

Figure 31 .1

Examination

She is normotensive and continues to slowly gain weight according to her antenatal records. She has widespread urticarial plaques over her palms, medial aspects of her arms, axillae, inner thighs and trunk (Fig. 31.1). There are two tense fluid-filled bullae overlying the erythema in her left axilla. There is no involvement of her mucous membranes. A recent fetal ultrasound scan confirmed her dates to be correct and did not identify any anomalies or abnormalities.

INVESTIGATIONS		
		Normal
Sodium	138 mmol/L	135–145 mmol/L
Potassium	3.6 mmol/L	3.5–5.0 mmol/L
Urea	5.2 mmol/L	2.5–6.7 mmol/L
Creatinine	61 μmol/L	70–120 μmol/L
Albumin	32 g/L	35–50 g/L
Glucose	5.8 mmol/L	4.0–6.0 mmol/L
Bilirubin	12 mmol/L	3–17 mmol/L
Alanine transaminase	18 IU/L	5–35 IU/L
Alkaline phosphatase	285 IU/L	30–300 IU/L
Urine dipstick	Negative for blood, leucocytes, protein, bilirubin, and glucose	

Questions

- What is this eruption and what are the possible differential diagnoses?
- How can you confirm the diagnosis?
- What is the management of this patient?

The clinical features in this case (specifically the distribution of the eruption and the presence of blisters) and the patient's history of a similar, possibly milder eruption occurring at a later stage of a previous pregnancy are highly suggestive of a diagnosis of pemphigoid gestationis (PG). Other differential diagnoses include pregnancy-specific dermatoses, primarily pruritic urticarial papules and plaques of pregnancy (a non-bullous eruption), and non-pregnancy associated eruptions (e.g. erythema multiforme, acute urticaria, scabies, allergic contact dermatitis, bullous pemphigoid, or other immunobullous diseases). Cholestasis of pregnancy is important to consider when faced with a pruritic patient in her mid-trimester without an eruption. It is associated with elevated serum bilirubin and a significant risk of fetal prematurity.

PG is a pregnancy-associated subepidermal immunobullous disease, analogous to bullous pemphigoid. The diagnosis can be confirmed by the demonstration of tissue-bound and circulating immunoglobulin G antibodies and complement, targeting the cutaneous basement membrane zone by direct and indirect immunofluorescence studies, and also by subepidermal blisters on histology.

There are several considerations when forming a management plan. First, the fetal outcome in PG is generally good; second, it is a self-limiting condition that is expected to remit following delivery (although it may occur earlier and in a more severe form during subsequent pregnancies). However, the intractable pruritus and associated blistering may lead to significant maternal morbidity. Superpotent topical steroids and systemic corticosteroids are used to control the eruption.

 KEY POINTS

- Pemphigoid gestationis (PG) is a pregnancy-associated subepidermal immunobullous disease analogous to bullous pemphigoid.
- PG presents with tense blisters overlying pruritic urticarial plaques.
- PG usually presents towards the end of the third trimester, however it may occur earlier and behave more aggressively in subsequent pregnancies.

History
A 31-year-old woman presents during the 35th week of her first pregnancy. She is very anxious about the development of extremely itchy 'lines' over her abdomen over the last two days. She is otherwise well with an unremarkable antenatal history to date. Her dates are confirmed on ultrasound scanning. She has no previous history of skin problems.

Examination
She has striking erythematous, linear, urticated lesions in a concentric and, in some areas, coalescing distribution over her pregnancy-distended abdomen (Fig. 32.1). The eruption corresponds with the striae distensae and there is sparing of the umbilicus. She has a few similar lesions over her upper thighs. She is normotensive and the remainder of her examination is normal. It is of note that according to her antenatal notes she has gained 5 kg since her last antenatal check 3 weeks ago. Urine dipstick is negative.

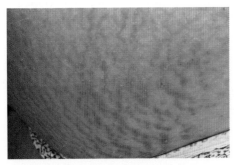

Figure 32.1

Questions
- What is this eruption?
- What other diagnoses would you consider?
- What are the implications for the baby?

This presentation with a very pruritic eruption beginning in the third trimester of the first pregnancy and arising within the striae distensae (sparing the umbilicus) is typical of pruritic urticarial papules and plaques of pregnancy (PUPPP), also referred to as toxic erythema of pregnancy or polymorphic eruption of pregnancy. Over a few days the eruption can become more widespread involving the trunk and extremities; less commonly, annular or polycyclic lesions develop. It is thought that maternal weight gain may somehow precipitate the lesions. Anecdotally it is more often associated with male fetus pregnancy and the risk of PUPPP seems to be higher with multiple gestation pregnancies.

It is important to consider other pregnancy-specific pruritic eruptions (such as pemphigoid gestationis, intrahepatic cholestasis of pregnancy) as well as common eruptions unrelated to pregnancy (such as urticaria, drug eruptions, viral exanthems, scabies). A comprehensive examination for evidence of scabies is indicated as well as investigations to rule out pemphigoid gestationis (skin biopsy for direct immunofluoresence studies).

Although PUPPP can be very symptomatic and consequently distressing for the affected mother, the eruption itself is not thought to have any adverse effects on the fetus. Management is therefore based on symptomatic relief with cool baths, light clothing, emollients and topical corticosteroids, as well as reassurance.

 KEY POINTS

- Pruritic urticarial papules and plaques of pregnancy (PUPPP) is a benign pregnancy dermatosis which usually arises in the third trimester.
- The most distressing aspect of the eruption is the associated pruritus. It is otherwise self-limited with no adverse effects on fetal outcome.
- The pathomechanism of the eruption is unknown but it is more commonly observed in association with recent, sudden weight gain, male fetus and multiple gestational pregnancies.

History

A 30-year-old woman presents with 10-month history of asymptomatic skin lesions developing over her trunk. Initially the lesions were red oval patches, which over many months became hard and the skin white. She does not have any joint problems, there is no family history of skin disease and she is otherwise well.

Examination

There are scattered, oval, indurated shiny white plaques with a purplish, poorly defined border predominantly over her trunk (Fig. 33.1). Some of the lesions have now become more hyperpigmented.

INVESTIGATIONS
Blood tests, skin biopsy.

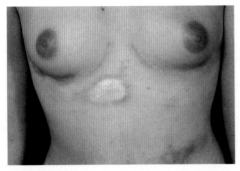

Figure 33.1

Questions

- What is the diagnosis?
- What are the possible triggers?
- How should the patient be managed?

This patient's skin biopsy confirmed the clinical diagnosis of morphoea. Palpation of the skin is an extremely important part of a dermatological examination. Plaques of morphoea feel very firm to the touch and the surface of the skin has lost its normal texture. The skin feels smooth and often waxy. Histopathology shows a proliferation of collagen in the dermis and subcutis. The cause of this localized dermal scleroderma is unknown. Women between the ages of 20–50 years are most commonly affected. The lesions themselves are usually asymptomatic. Skin changes are usually localized and initially erythematous/violaceous oval plaques which progress into ivory-coloured, hardening plaques measuring 1–20 cm in diameter. Morphoea may be circumscribed, generalized, linear and occasionally involve underlying structures (pansclerotic).

This patient had the generalized form of the disease with multiple plaques over her trunk. Linear morphoea, in contrast, normally affects the extremities, particularly over the frontoparietal scalp/face where a deep-seated form of linear scleroderma 'en coup de sabre' can occur. The sclerotic skin grows no hair and the underlying skull bone may become distorted.

Although the aetiology of morphoea is unknown, recognized triggers include local skin injury, post-radiation and viral infections such as measles. A small proportion of patients with classical morphoea developed the disease following tick bites, which transmit Lyme disease due to *Borrelia burgdorferi* infection. Autoantibodies may be positive including rheumatoid factor, antinuclear and antihistone antibodies.

The clinical course is generally slowly progressive, although some cases can 'burn out' and others spontaneously resolve. Extensive sclerotic plaques on the limbs can be associated with stiffness, weakness and loss of mobility.

Management is difficult. However, some success has been with topical vitamin D analogues (calcipotriol), intralesional and systemic corticosteroids, methotrexate, ciclosporin and psoralen–UVA/UVB or UVA1.

 KEY POINTS

- Morphoea appears as ivory-coloured, hardening plaques.
- It can be circumscribed, generalized, linear and may affect underlying structures.
- The aetiology is unknown, but triggers include local skin injury and viral infections.

History

A 54-year-old woman presents to the dermatology out-patient clinic with a two-year history of a gradual tightening of the skin over her fingers, forearms and legs. She also describes intermittent swelling of the hands and feet. Since her early 30s she had experienced pain in her digits on exposure to cold weather. Over the past few months she had noticed shortness of breath on exertion.

Examination

The skin over her fingers and hands appears oedematous, waxy, shiny, and indurated; normal skin elasticity has been lost. The distal fingers appear tapered and there is a small ulcer present on one of her finger pulps (Fig. 34.1). She has periorbital oedema and evidence of facial telangiectasia. On respiratory examination there are fine inspiratory crackles in the bilateral lower zone.

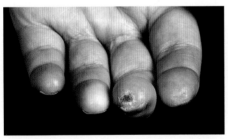

Figure 34.1

Questions

- What is the unifying diagnosis?
- Which organs may be involved?
- How should this patient be managed?

This patient was diagnosed with systemic sclerosis, which is a multisystem disease characterized by fibrotic and vascular abnormalities in association with autoimmune changes. This particularly affects the skin, lungs, heart and gastrointestinal tract.

The earliest skin changes are usually swelling of the hands and feet. Prior to this, however, patients may describe a long history of Raynaud's phenomenon, which is characterized by the fingers/toes undergoing a triphasic colour change from pallor (white), cyansois (blue) and rubor (red) following exposure to the cold. This occurs due to episodes of vasospasm, which causes peripheral vessels to constrict.

In association with intermittent hand and foot swelling are telangiectasia, which are visible dilated blood vessels occurring on the hands, face and chest. The hands have a characteristic appearance as in this patient including thickening of the skin over the fingers, which eventually leads to scarring (sclerosis). Fingers then become spindle-shaped with tapering, termed sclerodactyly, and feel tight and stiff. Skin tightening can result in difficulty opening the mouth (microstomia) and a 'beak-like' pinched appearance of the nose. Other late changes include finger pulp ulcers and even loss of digits.

This is a multisystem disorder affecting the gastrointestinal tract including oesophageal reflux, constipation, diarrhoea and malabsorption. Cardiorespiratory involvement includes pulmonary fibrosis and pericarditis. Renal involvement affects 50 per cent of patients. Joint and muscle pain occurs along with weakness and limited movement, resulting in contractures.

The diagnosis is generally made from the patient's clinical history and examination of the skin and other organs. Up to 90 per cent of patients have elevated antinuclear antibodies (ANA). Anticentromere antibodies are characteristic. Scl-70 is unique to systemic sclerosis and is more likely to be associated with severe systemic sclerosis involving the lungs.

Management of systemic sclerosis is challenging with as yet no cure. The course of this disease is progressive. Patients should be advised to keep their hands and feet warm with special warming gloves and fleecy boots. Vasodilating drugs and calcium channel blocking drugs may be beneficial. H2-blockers may reduce the gastrointestinal symptoms. Oral corticosteroids, cyclophosphamide and tacrolimus may be of benefit for limited periods. D-penicillamine may also help. Renal disease is the commonest cause of death, followed by cardiorespiratory disease.

 KEY POINTS

- Systemic sclerosis is a progressive, multisystem autoimmune disease.
- It particularly affects the skin, lungs, heart and gastrointestinal tract.
- There is no cure and so management is with supportive care.

History

A 23-year-old African Caribbean patient presents with an acute-onset facial rash. She has no rash elsewhere and no previous history of skin problems. She had taken an antihistamine for suspected allergy reaction as her face had become slightly swollen and red. Her family had become increasingly worried and took her to the local accident and emergency department. During her assessment she complained of a two-week history of general malaise, fatigue, fever and weight loss. On a systems review she admitted to having experienced intermittent joint pains involving her hands and knees.

Examination

She has a subtle erythematous confluent eruption present over her cheeks and nose which is ill-defined and slightly oedematous (Fig. 35.1); there is minimal scaling. The rest of her skin examination is normal including the scalp and nails, however she does have two ulcers present on her oral mucosa. She has tenderness in the small joints of her hands. Her temperature is 38.4 °C.

🔍 INVESTIGATIONS

		Normal
White cell count	6.4 × 10⁹/L	4.00–11.0 × 10⁹/L
Haemoglobin	10.9 g/dL	11.5–16.5 g/dL
Platelets	99 × 10⁹/L	150–450 × 10⁹/L
Neutrophils	4.92 × 10⁹/L	2.20–6.30 × 10⁹/L
Lymphocytes	0.9 × 10⁹/L	1.3–4.0 × 10⁹/L
Eosinophils	0.04 × 10⁹/L	0.00–0.40 × 10⁹/L
C-reactive protein	<5.0 mg/L	< 5 mg/L
Erythrocyte sedimentation rate (ESR)	35 mm/h	1–10 mm/h

Blood cultures were negative. A connective tissue screen was requested. Her ECG showed tachycardia. A skin biopsy was taken.

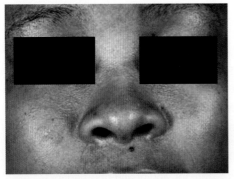

Figure 35.1

Questions

- What is the unifying diagnosis?
- What other cutaneous signs may be seen?
- Which other organ systems can be involved?

This type of clinical presentation can be a diagnostic challenge. Patients presenting with fever, malaise and weight loss may be suspected of suffering from systemic infections or malignancy. However, this patient had a facial rash and arthritis which should raise the possibility of a connective tissue disease. Consequently this patient was diagnosed with a serious multisystem autoimmune disease – namely systemic lupus erythematosus (SLE).

Patients with acute SLE classically develop a 'butterfly rash' over their cheeks and nose which is an erythematous, confluent, oedematous/macular eruption in the shape of a butterfly. Cutaneous lesions are found in 75 per cent of patients, including urticaria, bullae, photosensitivity, nailfold telangiectasia, calcinosis, vasculitis, Raynaud's phenomenon, diffuse/patchy alopecia and mouth ulcers. Patients may present acutely unwell with fever, weight loss and malaise. SLE is more common in women than men and is more common in African Caribbeans.

Multisystem involvement with serological or haematological abnormalities must be demonstrated to make the diagnosis of SLE within the framework of the revised American Rheumatism Association (ARA) criteria for the classification of SLE (see Table 35.1). Virtually any organ system can be affected by SLE including musculoskeletal (arthralgia, arthritis, myopathy) and renal, pericarditis, pneumonitis, hepatosplenomegaly, lymphadenopathy and peripheral neuropathies. Central nervous system (CNS) involvement can occur leading to seizures and psychiatric disturbances.

Table 35.1 **The diagnosis of SLE can be made if any 4 or more of the 11 criteria are present simultaneously or at any time during a patient's history**

	Criteria	Definition
1	Malar rash	Fixed erythema, flat or raised, over the malar eminences
2	Discoid rash	Erythematous circular raised patches with adherent keratotic scaling and follicular plugging; atrophic scarring may occur
3	Photosensitivity	Rash occurring following ultraviolet light exposure
4	Oral ulcers	Includes oral and nasopharyngeal ulcers, observed by doctor
5	Arthritis	Non-erosive arthritis of two or more peripheral joints, with tenderness, swelling, or effusion
6	Serositis	Pleuritis or pericarditis documented by ECG or rub or evidence of effusion
7	Renal disorder	Proteinuria > 0.5 g/d or 3+, or cellular casts
8	Neurological disorder	Seizures or psychosis without other causes
9	Haematological disorder	Haemolytic anemia or leucopenia (< 4000/L) or lymphopenia (< 1500/L) or thrombocytopenia (< 100 000/L) in the absence of offending drugs
10	Immunological disorder	Anti-dsDNA, anti-Sm, and/or anti-phospholipid
11	Antinuclear antibody	Abnormal ANA in the absence of drugs known to induce drug-induced lupus syndrome

Relevant investigations include a skin biopsy for histology and immunofluorescence where there is demonstration of IgG, IgM and C3 in a band-like pattern along the dermal–epidermal junction. Anti-nuclear antibodies (ANA) are positive in over 90 per cent of cases. Further positive autoantibodies including anti-double strand DNA and extractable nuclear antigen, anticardiolipin autoantiboides (lupus anticoagulant) may also be seen. Blood tests may also reveal a normocytic, normochromic anaemia, lymphopenia, thrombocytopenia, raised ESR and low complement levels. Patients should be investigated for any concurrent infections to which they are susceptible.

Management of SLE during an acute attack can be challenging. Patients often need admission to hospital for rest, investigations and systemic corticosteroids. If there is obvious renal and CNS involvement or significant systemic upset, then high-dose pulsed methylprednisolone may be required. When patients are stable they should be advised about photoprotection. Long-term management may include hydroxychloroquine for cutaneous disease and steroid-sparing immunosuppressants such as azathioprine, mycophenolate mofetil and cyclophosphamide.

KEY POINTS

- Systemic lupus erythematosus (SLE) is a serious multisystem autoimmune disease affecting mainly females.
- Clinical presentations of acute SLE may be misdiagnosed as infections/malignancy.
- Cutaneous lesions are found in 75 per cent of patients with SLE.

History

A 39-year-old patient presents to her GP with a rash of fairly sudden onset, which initially affected her chest and arms and then spread to her back. She had noticed that the eruption started as small red spots that were dry and scaly, which then spread out in a ring-shape. She was worried she might have caught ring-worm in the school where she works. However, it seemed to start after her recent holiday in Spain. The rash is asymptomatic. She has no previous history of skin problems, and is otherwise well.

Examination

There is an erythematous eruption predominantly affecting her face, neck, trunk and proximal limbs. The lesions are annular in appearance, sharply defined with an overlying surface scale. The lesions display central regression and coalesce to give a polycyclic appearance (Fig. 36.1). Her scalp nails and mucosae are normal.

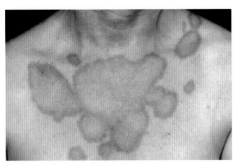

Figure 36.1

Questions

- What is the cutaneous diagnosis?
- What systemic manifestations may be associated?
- How should this patient be managed?

This patient presented with the classic skin eruption of subacute cutaneous lupus erythematosus (SCLE). The rash appears fairly suddenly, especially over sun-exposed sites, and is symmetrical and scaly. There are characteristically bright red, annular, well-demarcated lesions with central regression. Overlying the erythema there is an almost psorisiform scale. The eruption mainly affects the upper trunk (shoulders and 'V' of the chest) and dorsi of the hands (sun-exposed sites). SCLE occurs in young and middle-aged patients and is more common in females. It is usually a very persistent eruption lasting many months.

Approximately 50 per cent of patients will also meet a few of the criteria for systemic lupus erythematosus (SLE) as defined by the American Rheumatism Association (see also Table 35.1). These mainly include photosensitivity, arthralgia, serositis and serologic abnormalities. The serious organ involvement of SLE is uncommon, although renal and CNS involvement can rarely occur and thus all SCLE patients should be investigated for systemic disease.

Virtually all patients with SCLE have circulating anti-Ro (SS-A) and 30–50 per cent will have anti-La antibodies. Pregnant women with Ro (SS-A) positive SCLE may give birth to babies with neonatal lupus due to placental transfer. The rash is morphologically similar to SCLE, but is transient. More seriously, congenital heart block can occur. The heart block is usually permanent requiring a pacemaker and all women of child-bearing age should be counselled accordingly. Coexistent Sjörgren's syndrome with SCLE has been reported.

A comprehensive drug history is essential in patients with SCLE, as the disease can be triggered by certain medications including naproxen, nifedipine, verapamil, diltiazem and terbinafine.

Cutaneous disease is most often the commonest concern of patients. Sun avoidance and photoprotection are essential in all patients. Some patients do respond to potent topical corticosteroids, but many require systemic therapy to control the cutaneous disease, including thalidomide and hydroxychloroquine. A small proportion of patients may go on to develop SLE.

 KEY POINTS

- The rash of subacute cutaneous lupus erythematosus (SCLE) characteristically displays erythematous annular lesions with central regression.
- 50 per cent of patients with SCLE will also have a few of the criteria of SLE.
- Virtually all patients with SCLE have circulating anti-Ro (SS-A) antibodies.

History

A 55-year-old woman presents to the dermatology clinic with a long history of a rash that occurred during the spring and summer months over her face and scalp. Over the past few years the affected area became more extensive, the skin became scarred and she noticed her hair did not grow back. She wears a hair weave to cover the area. More recently, however, she has developed new lesions over her cheeks and is worried about scarring. She is otherwise well.

Examination

There are large areas of scarring with associated hypo- and hyperpigmentation. She has alopecia predominantly over her fronto-temporal scalp (Fig. 37.1). Over the face and vertex of the scalp there are indurated erythematous plaques with overlying scale and follicular plugging. Her ears are similarly affected. Full skin examination was otherwise normal as were her nails.

INVESTIGATIONS
A skin biopsy was performed.

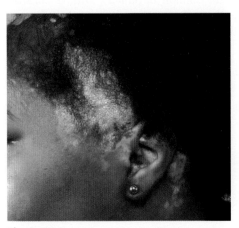

Figure 37.1

Questions

- What is the diagnosis?
- What other investigations might you arrange?

The scalp shows areas of alopecia with skin atrophy and scarring in the affected areas. These changes are typical of discoid lupus erythematosus (DLE), which is a chronic, persistent, often indolent disorder seen mainly in women. DLE is characterized by fixed, indurated, erythematous plaques with overlying scale, predominantly over the face and scalp. The plaques in DLE are often annular or polycyclic and well demarcated. As the lesions expand, central regression occurs and, unlike in subacute cutaneous lupus erythematosus (SCLE), atrophy and eventually significant scarring results. 'Burned out' lesions become pink or hypopigmented but in Asian and African Caribbean patients the skin may also show hyperpigmentation. Permanently scarring alopecia is often a common feature which can be very disfiguring. The external auditory canals are frequently involved as in this patient.

A skin biopsy in DLE revealed hyperkeratosis, epidermal atrophy, follicular plugging and degeneration of the basal cell layer. A perifollicular lymphocytic inflammatory infiltrate was seen. A positive immunofluorescence was seen in more than 85 per cent of new lesions.

Patients should be screened for systemic lupus erythematosus (SLE) with a full blood count, liver and kidney function tests, clotting time and auto-antibody titre. If the initial work-up does not reveal systemic involvement the risk of developing SLE is only 1–5 per cent. Lesions of DLE are, however, not uncommon in patients with established SLE and can be found in up to 25 per cent of patients during the course of their disease. Complete remission occurs in 40 per cent of all patients.

DLE without intervention can persist for many years and lead to extensive scarring. Early diagnosis and treatment are therefore essential to prevent further scarring. The mainstay of treatment is with photoprotection (SPF > 30). Potent topical corticosteroids can be very effective for active lesions. Antimalarials, gold and other immunosuppressants may be required.

 KEY POINTS

- Without treatment discoid lupus erythematosus (DLE) can result in permanent scarring and disfiguring alopecia on the scalp.
- Screening for systemic disease should be undertaken. which occurs in 1–5 per cent of patients with DLE.
- Rigorous photoprotection is advised to try to prevent further DLE lesions appearing.

History

A 59-year-old woman visited her GP as she was concerned about unexplained weight loss. Her GP noted an erythematous rash around her eyes and over the dorsum of her hands and referred her to the dermatology clinic. On direct questioning she does complain about difficulty in getting up out of a chair and climbing the stairs. She denies any other symptoms apart from a persistent dry cough. She is a life-long smoker and drinks alcohol socially.

Examination

She has erythematous flattish papules over the extensor surfaces of her interphalangeal and metacarpal phalangeal joints (Fig. 38.1). In the periorbital region she has a violaceous erythema with subtle oedema (Fig. 38.2). There is an erythematous non-scaly macular rash affecting her neck and upper back. Neurological examination reveals proximal limb weakness.

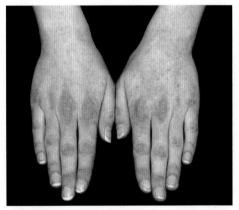

Figure 38.1

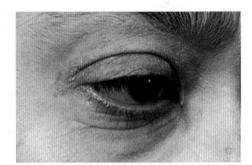

Figure 38.2

Questions

- What is the cutaneous diagnosis?
- What may be the underlying condition?
- How should this patient be managed?

The cutaneous manifestations of this disease may be striking or more subtle; therefore a high index of clinical suspicion is needed to make the diagnosis of dermatomyositis. The erythematous, purplish, flat papules over the extensor surfaces of the interphalangeal joints are termed Gottron's papules and are pathognomonic of dermatomyositis. The periorbital heliotrope rash with associated oedema is also highly suggestive of the diagnosis. Erythema around the posterior and 'V' of the neck is the so-called Shawl's sign. Periungal erythema with telangiectasia may also be classically seen.

Muscle involvement is usually manifest by muscle tenderness and weakness with a proximal myopathy. Patients will describe difficulty rising from a supine position, climbing the stairs or combing their hair. In some cases muscle involvement of the bulbar, pharyngeal and oesophageal areas can occur leading to difficulty in breathing and swallowing. Muscle involvement may precede, follow or occur simultaneously with cutaneous disease.

Dermatomyositis is rare and the cause remains unknown. However, a high proportion of affected patients over the age of 50 years had an associated underlying malignancy. This patient was a smoker with weight loss and, following further investigations, was diagnosed with a carcinoma of the bronchus. The most common types of malignancies associated with dermatomyositis involve the ovary, breast, lung and gastrointestinal tract.

A skin biopsy may be helpful but histopathology is not specific to dermatomyositis. Raised muscle enzymes are typically seen including creatine kinase and lactate dehydrogenase. Non-specific antinuclear antibodies (ANA) are found in most patients, specific anti-Mi-1 is found in around 25 per cent and anti-Jo-1 in just a few. An electromyogram of an affected muscle will generally be abnormal and biopsy of an affected muscle can also be helpful. Magnetic resonance imaging is often the preferred investigation, if available, to show focal muscle involvement.

A moderate to high dose of oral corticosteroids is usually the initial therapy given. Steroid sparing agents used in the second line include methotrexate, azathioprine, ciclosporin, mycophenolate, cyclophosphamide and high-dose intravenous immunoglobulin. The prognosis in most patients is relatively good except in those with respiratory myopathy or with an underlying malignancy. A better prognosis is seen in individuals who receive early immunosuppression. Most patients will require treatment for life; however, in about 20 per cent of patients the condition abates. Patients are advised to avoid excessive sun exposure and to use photoprotective measures. Patients should be followed up and screened regularly for the possibility of underlying malignancy which may reveal itself in time.

 KEY POINTS

- Gottron's papules are pathognomonic of dermatomyositis.
- An underlying malignancy should be excluded in older patients.
- Early intervention with immunosuppression leads to a better prognosis.

History

A 24-year-old fashion design student presents to the accident and emergency department with a 1-week history of feeling unwell with a temperature, abdominal pain, diarrhoea and headaches. Overnight he has developed a widespread asymptomatic rash, mainly over his face and trunk. His college friend was worried about him and brought him to the hospital. The patient reports being previously well although he admitted to having a penile discharge a few weeks previously that had settled spontaneously. He has not travelled outside the UK for at least 5 years. He takes no prescription medication but takes occasional vitamin supplements.

Examination

Multiple small erythematous macules and papules were seen over the patient's face, neck and trunk (Fig. 39.1), with scattered lesions on his limbs. Conjunctivae were unaffected; he had a slightly 'coated' tongue but no ulceration in his mouth. Genital examination was normal. He had shotty lymphadenopathy in the cervical region.

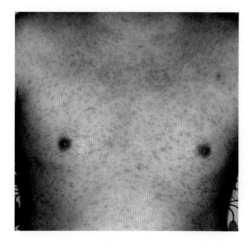

Figure 39.1

Questions

- What investigations would you request?
- What is your differential diagnosis?
- What diagnosis do you suspect and how would you treat him?

Widespread erythematous maculopapular rashes are a sign of a 'reactive' process and are usually caused by 'drugs or bugs'. Antibiotics, NSAIDs, anticonvulsants and thiazide diuretics are amongst the most common medications to result in these eruptions, termed toxic erythema. Viral infections such as measles, Epstein–Barr virus (glandular fever), influenzae infections and acute viral hepatitis may also present with 'flu-like' symptoms and this type of non-specific skin eruption.

This patient was diagnosed with a primary human immunodeficiency virus infection (HIV-seroconversion). Approximately 4 weeks after becoming infected with HIV it is estimated that 70–90 per cent of patients develop symptoms that may include general malaise, headache, sore throat, fever, abdominal pain and diarrhoea. Sixty per cent of patients develop an asymptomatic classically morbilliform rash with erythematous macules and papules mainly on the face, neck and trunk. Mouth or genital ulcers may also be present.

A high index of clinical suspicion is needed to make the diagnosis of primary HIV infection as the rash and the symptoms are non-specific. A detailed history of potential risk factors should be undertaken. Symptoms of primary HIV usually start within 4 weeks of a high-risk exposure. Known risk factors include originating from an endemic area, intravenous drug users who share needles, men who have sex with men, sex workers, people with multiple sexual partners and unprotected sexual intercourse. Vertical transmission from HIV-infected women to the fetus *in utero* is also a route of spread.

Patients should give consent for an HIV test to look for viral antigen (usually detectable by day 8 using PCR techniques) as well as antibodies (detectable by weeks 2–4). Full blood count may show a lymphopenia and a low CD4 count is frequently seen on T-cell subset analysis.

Treating primary HIV infection with antiretroviral medication is controversial. At present most doctors feel commencement of highly active antiretroviral treatment (HAART) at the time of HIV seroconversion is optional. Many patients presenting at this stage of the disease are being enrolled into large multi-centre trials to see if HAART is effective or not in the short or long term. There is an increasing body of evidence, however, which suggests that HAART may need to be started when the CD4 count drops below 350 cells/µL, rather than 200 cells/µL as was previously thought.

 KEY POINTS

- Primary HIV infection presents with non-specific flu-like symptoms and a maculopapular rash.
- A high index of suspicion and arranging appropriate serological tests are essential to make the diagnosis.
- Always think 'could this be a primary HIV infection?' when you see patients with a reactive rash.

History

A 23-year-old African Caribbean man presents with a 2-year history of gradual patchy lightening of the skin. He denies any symptoms such as itching or irritation of his skin prior to the onset of the whitening patches. He has no previous history of skin problems but had suffered with mild asthma as a child. He is otherwise well and does not take medication. There is a family history of thyroid disease.

Examination

There are multiple, well-demarcated, non-scaly macules of depigmentation in a symmetrical distribution, predominantly over the trunk (Fig. 40.1). The periorbital, perioral and genital areas are also affected. Some of the macules have tiny pigmented spots within them.

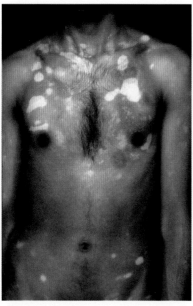

Figure 40.1

Questions

- What is the diagnosis?
- What are the different presentations of this disease?
- How should this patient be managed?

This patient presented with depigmentation (leucoderma) which was asymptomatic and symmetrical. Causes of hypopigmentation include albinism, hypopituitarism, chemical leucoderma such as with phenolics, and post-inflammatory change secondary to inflammatory dermatoses such as eczema. Onset in this patient was in adulthood (acquired) with gradual deterioration, which led to the diagnosis of vitiligo.

Vitiligo is a depigmenting acquired disease that occurs due to loss of epidermal melanocytes. Vitiligo has been reported to be associated with autoimmune disease including thyroid disease, pernicious anaemia and type 1 diabetes mellitus. The cause of vitiligo is, however, unknown. It affects 1 per cent of the population, usually occurring between the ages of 10 and 30 years. Vitiligo affects all racial groups, but is particularly distressing in those with darker skin.

Vitiligo is characterized by sharply defined pale/white macules. Most commonly affected are periorbital, perioral and anogenital areas, but also the axillae, inguinal regions and extensor sites of the knees/elbows. Symmetrical involvement is the norm. In addition, white hair and prematurely grey hair can occur.

There are several types: a focal type which is characterized by one or more macules; segmental vitiligo occurs when the disease develops unilaterally, for instance, down one leg; generalized or universal disease can also occur. In patients with lighter skin where the contrast between disease and normal skin is less obvious, then a Wood's light can be very helpful to evaluate the macules.

The course of vitiligo is variable; however, most patients' course is quite rapid at the onset followed by a period of stability. Treatments are generally unsatisfactory. Photoprotective advice is essential for involved skin. Cosmetic camouflage can be useful. To induce repigmentation, topical corticosteroids and topical calcineurin inhibitors such as tacrolimus can be effective for focal lesions. For more extensive disease phototherapy including psoralen–UVA and narrow-band UVB are effective in some patients. Response to phototherapy is usually evidenced initially by follicular repigmentation where tiny macular dots of pigmented skin are seen. In extensive disease, patients may be offered depigmentation of their remaining normal skin using monobezyl ether or hydroquinone.

 KEY POINTS

- Vitiligo occurs due to loss of epidermal melanocytes.
- It has been reported to be associated with autoimmune disease.
- Focal, segmental and generalized types exist.

History

A 23-year-old woman visits the GP practice nurse because of persistently high blood pressure. During the course of her discussion she mentions incidentally that she is cosmetically troubled by 'lumps' on her skin, which leads the nurse to refer her to the dermatology clinic. She describes the lumps as asymptomatic but gradually accumulating, particularly over her trunk. She is otherwise well and on no medication. Her parents and sister are also well with no history of hypertension, coronary artery disease or similar skin lesions.

Examination

On examination, her blood pressure is 170/110 mmHg. She has an unusual pigmentary pattern with generalized freckling or lentigines affecting non–sun-exposed sites (such as inframammary, axillae and groin) as well as sun-exposed sites. She has scattered tan-coloured macules over her trunk and proximal legs (12 in total); these macules vary in size, but have a regular shape and borders (Fig. 41.1). She also has soft, fleshy, non-tender, pink to skin-coloured smooth nodules, some of which protrude and are pedunculated and some are located deeper within the dermis. She has normal heart sounds, but she does have a clearly audible right-sided abdominal bruit. The remainder of her examination is normal.

INVESTIGATIONS		
		Normal
Haemoglobin	12.5 g/dL	13.3–17.7 g/dL
Mean corpuscular volume	91 fL	80–99 fL
White cell count	8.2×10^9/L	$3.9–10.6 \times 10^9$/L
Platelets	400×10^9/L	$150–440 \times 10^9$/L
Sodium	138 mmol/L	135–145 mmol/L
Potassium	4.2 mmol/L	3.5–5.0 mmol/L
Urea	5.5 mmol/L	2.5–6.7 mmol/L
Creatinine	82 µmol/L	70–120 µmol/L
Albumin	36 g/L	35–50 g/L
Glucose	4.2 mmol/L	4.0–6.0 mmol/L

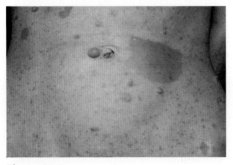

Figure 41.1

Questions

- What is the diagnosis?
- How should this patient be further investigated?
- What genetic counselling should she receive?

The dermatological features (cutaneous neurofibromas with axillary, groin and submammary freckling) are pathognomonic of neurofibromatosis type 1 (NF1). Other cutaneous features of NF1 include hypopigmented macules, cutaneous angiomas, transient xanthogranulomas and glomus tumours. She has associated hypertension, and the presence of a unilateral bruit is suggestive of renal artery stenosis, a recognized complication of NF1.

Further investigations are not required to confirm a diagnosis of NF1. Molecular testing can be considered, and the causative mutation in the *NF1* gene can be detected in 95 per cent of cases, but there is not as yet a well-defined genotype–phenotype correlation. Imaging studies to look for central nervous system or bony features of NF1 can be performed if symptomatic. There is no medical indication to excise the cutaneous neurofibromas as, unlike subcutaneous or plexiform neurofibromas, they are not associated with malignant transformation. They can be a source of psychological distress.

The priority for this patient is to identify the cause of her high blood pressure and initiate appropriate treatment. High blood pressure in NF1 can be a primary process or may be secondary to other NF1 complications, such as renal artery stenosis or phaeochromocytoma. This patient should have urgent assessment for renal artery stenosis (including duplex ultrasonography) and 24-hour urinary catecholamine collection to rule out phaeochromocytoma. It is reassuring that her renal function is normal on routine biochemistry, but a protein/creatinine ratio on a random void urine specimen should be performed to assess the level of renal dysfunction and identify any mild to moderate proteinuria which is frequently seen in association with renal vascular disease.

NF1 is an autosomal dominant disorder and the responsible gene is located on chromosome 17. Its protein product, called neurofibromin, is widely expressed particularly in the nervous system. Mutations in the *NF1* gene predispose to tumour formation. Formal genetic counselling would be advised before this patient plans pregnancy; she should be informed of a 50 per cent risk of transmitting NF1 to each offspring. The complications of NF1 vary between individuals and are unpredictable within families; there is a 1 in 12 risk for this patient of having a severely affected child. Where a pathogenic *NF1* mutation is known, both prenatal testing and pre-implantation genetic diagnosis are available. Approximately 50 per cent of affected individuals have new mutations, however the family of this patient should be examined for any suggestive features.

! The seven diagnostic criteria for NF1 (at least two are required for diagnosis, however many do not appear until adolescence)

- Six or more café-au-lait spots or hyperpigmented macules ≥ 5 mm in diameter in children younger than 10 years and to 15 mm in adults
- Axillary or inguinal freckles
- Two or more typical neurofibromas or one plexiform neurofibroma
- Optic nerve glioma
- Two or more iris hamartomas (Lisch nodules), often identified only through slit-lamp examination by an ophthalmologist
- Sphenoid dysplasia or typical long-bone abnormalities such as pseudarthrosis
- First-degree relative (e.g. mother, father, sister, brother) with NF1

Café au lait macules (CALMs) and their significance

- If 1 CALM – no significance
- If > 3 CALMs in Caucasian – follow-up for development of multiple system disease
- If > 5 CALMs – monitor closely for NF-1
- If other additional features, such as bone fractures or precocious puberty associated with a large CALM or Blashkoid hyperpigmentation (McCune–Albright syndrome) consider referral to clinical geneticist
- Other conditions associated with CALMs include NF2, McCune–Albright syndrome, and Legius syndrome

KEY POINTS

- Neurofibromatosis type 1 (NF1) is an autosomal dominantly inherited multisystem condition with major skin features and many potential clinical complications.
- Periodic blood pressure monitoring is part of the routine surveillance of an affected individual.
- Cutaneous features of NF1 include café au lait macules, axillary and groin freckling, neurofibromas, hypomelanotic macules, xanthogranulomas, angiomas and glomus tumours.

History

A 13-year-old girl attends your clinic with her mother. She is complaining of skin changes affecting her neck, which have been progressively worsening over the past 18 months. In particular the changes are leading to name-calling at school with her peers saying her neck is 'dirty'. Her school attendance for the last term was only 87 per cent.

She is a very quiet girl and there is little eye contact through the consultation. Both she and her mother acknowledge that she is overweight. Her menarche was at the age of 11 years and 3 months, her menses are irregular. She is not on medication. She is an only child. Her mother has type 2 diabetes, hypertension and is also overweight, her father suffers from asthma.

Examination

Her height is 163 cm and weight 97.5 kg – a body mass index (BMI) of 37 – and blood pressure 140/85 mmHg. She has symmetrical hyperpigmented velvety thickened papillomatous plaques associated with scattered skin tags (acrochordons) around her neck, especially posteriorly and laterally, as well as in her axillae (Fig. 42.1) and groin (intertriginous sites). She has mild to moderately severe comedonal acne over face and chest. There are longitudinal striae over her lower abdomen and thighs. There is no evidence of hirsutism.

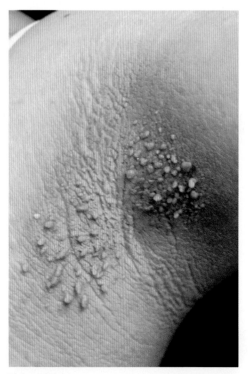

Figure 42.1

Questions

- What is the problem affecting this patient's neck and axillae?
- What is the likely underlying pathogenesis?
- What complications might you consider?

The hyperpigmented, velvety thickening of the skin in the intertriginous zones, including this patient's neck and axillae, represent acanthosis nigricans, usually a clinical diagnosis which very rarely requires histological confirmation. It often coexists with acrochordons. It is thought to be caused by factors that stimulate epidermal keratinocyte and dermal fibroblast proliferation. The most common association with acanthosis nigricans in young patients is insulin resistance. In older patients with new-onset acanthosis nigricans, an associated (usually aggressive) internal malignancy (particularly gastrointestinal) must be considered. Familial and syndromic forms of acanthosis nigricans have also been identified. Many syndromes share common features, including obesity, hyperinsulinaemia and craniosynostosis.

The definition of childhood obesity depends on age-dependent centile charts, however a BMI of > 30 kg/m^2 is generally accepted as obese. The unfortunate complications of childhood obesity are manifold. It predisposes to insulin resistance and type 2 diabetes, hypertension, hyperlipidaemia, liver and renal disease, reproductive dysfunction and orthopaedic problems. It also increases the risk of adult-onset obesity and cardiovascular disease. Emotional and psychosocial sequelae are widespread. Anecdotal evidence suggests that depression and eating disorders are common in children and adolescents referred to obesity clinics. Prejudice and discrimination against individuals with obesity are ubiquitous within youth culture; even very young children have been found to regard their peers who have obesity in negative ways. Social isolation, peer problems, and lower self-esteem are frequently observed. The presence of acanthosis nigricans is an important predictor of metabolic syndrome of insulin resistance and polycystic ovary syndrome in later life unless the BMI is addressed.

Acanthosis nigricans is not a skin disease per se, but rather a sign of an underlying problem. If associated with insulin resistance, the most common cause, treatment of the metabolic abnormality may lead to improvement of the appearance of the skin. Dietary changes and weight loss may cause the acanthosis nigricans to regress almost completely.

! Investigation of a patient with acanthosis nigricans

- Oral glucose tolerance test
- Fasting lipid panel for detection of dyslipidaemia
- Thyroid function tests
- Karyotype
- Growth hormone secretion and function tests, when indicated
- Assessment of reproductive hormones (including prolactin), when indicated
- For older patients with new-onset acanthosis nigricans: work-up for occult malignancy

---

KEY POINTS

- Acanthosis nigricans is a marker of underlying medical disorders, most commonly linked with insulin resistance, although amongst older patients acanthosis nigricans may occur as a paraneoplastic phenomenon.
- Identification and treatment of the underlying disorder will improve the appearance of the skin changes.
- In addition this patient's striae and acne may respond to weight loss.

History

A 26-year-old woman is referred by the orthopaedic surgeons for an urgent dermatology opinion. Three weeks previously she had sustained a lower leg laceration at work and had attended the accident and emergency department where the wound was cleaned and sutured. Within four days the sutures had dehisced, so she presented to her GP who prescribed a course of flucloxacillin. Two days later, with an enlarging ulcer and increasing pain, she attended the A&E once more. The concern was of potential extending necrotic infection, such as necrotizing fasciitis and she was taken to theatre for urgent debridement and commenced on intravenous vancomycin and gentamicin. In theatre the ulcer was debrided but the base, surrounding skin and fascia were all noted to be healthy. She continued on antibiotics and daily ulcer dressing. There was no growth from any of the swabs or samples sent for microbiological, atypical mycobacterial, viral or mycological analysis. Over the next 10 days the ulcerated areas have continued to extend associated with extreme pain. She also complains of lethargy and arthralgia. She is a non-smoker and is otherwise well. She has no past medical history.

Examination

There is marked erythema and swelling of the distal third of the right lower leg, ankle and proximal foot. There are two areas of ulceration: a smaller regularly shaped ulcer anteromedially, and a more irregularly shaped and larger ulcer extending posteriorly from the medial malleolus (Fig. 43.1). Both have raised, purple to red inflammatory borders. The bases of the ulcers are covered with adherent yellow slough. The surrounding skin (particularly distal to the ulceration) is erythematous and there is marked swelling. Pedal pulses are difficult to palpate on the affected side due to pain and swelling, however bedside Doppler studies confirm good flow.

🔍 INVESTIGATIONS		
		Normal
Haemoglobin	10.4 g/dL	13.3–17.7 g/dL
Mean corpuscular volume	87 fL	80–99 fL
White cell count	22.6 × 10⁹/L	3.9–10.6 × 10⁹/L
Platelets	633 × 10⁹/L	150–440 × 10⁹/L
Erythrocyte sedimentation rate	98 mm/h	< 10 mm/h
C-reactive protein	22 mg/L	< 5 mg/L

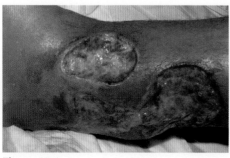

Figure 43.1

Questions

- What are these lesions?
- How can the diagnosis be confirmed?
- What is the management of this patient?

This presentation is not typical of many types of leg ulceration; both venous and arterial ulceration are easily excluded. The history of a penetrating injury followed by an enlarging wound and pain must raise the concern of infection and/or foreign body reaction. Necrotizing fasciitis is a progressive, rapidly spreading, inflammatory infection located in the deep fascia, with secondary necrosis of the subcutaneous tissues. It can be difficult to recognize in its early stage, but without aggressive treatment is associated with a high mortality and morbidity even amongst previously fit and healthy individuals. Other infective differential diagnoses include ecthyma (an ulcerative pyoderma of the skin caused by group A β-haemolytic Streptococci) and sporotrichosis (a subcutaneous or systemic infection caused by *Sporothrix schenckii*, a rapidly growing dimorphic fungus). Cultures in this circumstance should be continued for at least six weeks before being declared negative.

The lack of positive culture despite provision of surgically obtained affected tissue samples, as well as the lack of response to broad-spectrum systemic antimicrobial agents, makes infection unlikely. The clinical features would be consistent with the presentation of pyoderma gangrenosum. The diagnosis of pyoderma gangrenosum is one of exclusion, histopathological features can include massive neutrophilic infiltration, haemorrhage, and necrosis of the overlying epidermis; however, they are non-specific. Approximately 50 per cent of patients with pyoderma gangrenosum have an underlying systemic disease such as inflammatory bowel disease, myelodysplasia, lupus or other autoimmune diseases. Full systemic work-up to exclude these conditions is essential, as treatment of the underlying disorder may improve the cutaneous features.

Treatment of pyoderma gangrenosum can be challenging. Surgery should be avoided, if possible, because of the pathergic phenomenon that may occur with surgical manipulation or grafting, resulting in wound enlargement. Topical therapies include gentle local wound care and dressings, superpotent topical corticosteroids and antiseptic precautions. Systemic immunosuppression with agents such as corticosteroids, ciclosporin, mycophenolate mofetil, cyclophosphamide, anti-tumour necrosis factor agents such infliximab and even intravenous immunoglobulins are used. Adequate pain relief is crucial.

 KEY POINTS

- Pyoderma gangrenosum is an uncommon ulcerative cutaneous condition of uncertain aetiology. Ulcerations of pyoderma gangrenosum may occur after trauma or injury to the skin in 30 per cent of patients; this process is termed pathergy.
- The diagnosis is made by excluding other causes of similar appearing cutaneous ulcerations, including infection, malignancy, vasculitis, collagen vascular diseases, diabetes and trauma.
- Therapy of pyoderma gangrenosum involves the use of anti-inflammatory agents, such as corticosteroids, and immunosuppressive agents.

History

A 23-year-old woman attends the dermatology clinic complaining of the appearance of asymptomatic lesions on her legs. She has a background of type 1 diabetes mellitus, diagnosed at age 6 years. Her glycaemic control had been erratic when she first moved to university 4 years ago, however she now feels more in control of her glucose levels with careful titration of her insulin.

Examination

There are bilateral skin lesions affecting her anterior shins. The individual lesions are discrete and well demarcated with irregular borders. There is atrophy of the dermis and epidermis resulting in a shiny (but 'transparent') surface with yellow colour and apparent arborizing telangiectasia (Fig. 44.1). A full examination including fundoscopy was otherwise unremarkable. She has no skin lesions elsewhere.

INVESTIGATIONS		
		Normal
Haemoglobin	13.8 g/dL	13.3–17.7 g/dL
Mean corpuscular volume	93 fL	80–99 fL
White cell count	7.9 × 10⁹/L	3.9–10.6 × 10⁹/L
Platelets	431 × 10⁹/L	150–440 × 10⁹/L
Sodium	136 mmol/L	135–145 mmol/L
Potassium	4.2 mmol/L	3.5–5.0 mmol/L
Urea	8.5 mmol/L	2.5–6.7 mmol/L
Creatinine	58 µmol/L	70–120 µmol/L
Albumin	38 g/L	35–50 g/L
Bilirubin	15 µmol/L	3–17 µmol/L
Alanine transaminase	29 IU/L	5–35 IU/L
Alkaline phosphatase	126 IU/L	30–300 IU/L
HbA1C	8.5%	6.5–7.5%
Urinalysis	Negative for blood; 1+ for protein; negative for leucocytes	

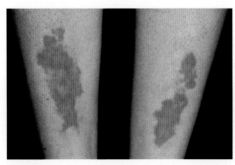

Figure 44.1

Questions

- What are these lesions?
- What complications can be associated with them?
- How would you manage this patient?

This patient has a history of poor glycaemic control and evidence of diabetic nephropathy. Her current HbA1c value is acceptable but could be tighter. These skin lesions are called necrobiosis lipoidica (NL), which is associated with diabetes mellitus, particularly type 1. The frequency of diabetes mellitus amongst patients with NL ranges from 10 to 70 per cent in various studies, and the prevalence of NL amongst patients with diabetes mellitus ranges from 0.3 to 3.0 per cent. The association with poor glycaemic control is controversial. However, exercise and improved glycaemic control are reported to improve the lesions. The lesions initially present as red/brown papules and nodules which may resemble granuloma annulare or cutaneous sarcoid. They gradually flatten and become atrophic, taking on the characteristic appearance seen in Figure 44.1. NL has a predilection for the anterior shins, but may also occur elsewhere on the lower legs and feet.

Although the clinical course may be indolent, NL lesions can be associated with refractory ulceration. The clinical appearance and lack of spontaneous remission often prompts therapeutic intervention. Treatment of NL can be disappointing. Once established the hallmark of these lesions is atrophy and few therapeutic interventions improve their appearance. Early application of topical glucocorticoids may slow progression. Some authors advocate intralesional glucocorticoid injections, but these carry an associated risk of ulceration. Other treatment modalities described include phototherapy with psoralen–UVA and even aspirin. Ulcerated NL is managed with dressings and immunosuppressive therapy (ciclosporin, methotrexate and systemic glucocorticoids).

❗ Cutaneous complications of diabetes mellitus

- Acanthosis nigricans
- Necrobiosis lipoidica
- Sceleroderma-like syndrome (limited mobility around small joints, especially hands)
- Scleredema – painless insidious induration and thickening of skin over the upper back, shoulders and neck
- Granuloma annulare – weak association with diabetes mellitus
- Eruptive xanthomas – reddish-yellow papules over the buttocks and extensor surfaces of extremities, associated with severe underlying hypertriglyceridaemia
- Cutaneous infections – bacterial (e.g. cellulitis, erysipelas), fungal
- Diabetic ulcers
- Bullosis diabeticorum
- Lipodystrophy – following subcutaneous administration of insulin

---

KEY POINTS

- Necrobiosis lipoidica (NL) is characterized by discrete atrophic shiny yellow patches with telangiectasis over the anterior shins.
- It can be associated with diabetes mellitus.
- The challenging aspects of NL include the cosmetic impact as well as lack of effective therapeutic modality.
- Ulceration is the most serious complication.

History

A 51-year-old man presents to his GP with progressive swelling of the lower legs. He works as a teacher and had initially ignored the changes, assuming they resulted from standing all day. However, the swelling did not recede overnight and his shins were becoming 'lumpy'. He feels otherwise well in himself, reporting plenty of 'energy' in the classroom, although he has lost weight recently which he can't explain. There is a family history of varicose veins and diabetes. He takes occasional paracetamol for headaches and 'tired eyes' at the end of the day.

Examination

There are bilateral pigmented plaques of the anterior shins, worse on the left than the right, and the associated swelling does not pit on firm pressure (Fig. 45.1). There is no evidence of varicose veins. He has mild proptosis and clubbing, and is of slim build. There is no obvious swelling in his neck. His scalp and nails are normal.

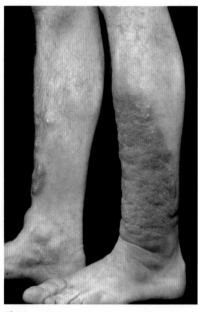

Figure 45.1

Questions

- What investigations would you request?
- What is the diagnosis?
- How would you manage this patient?

One of the many exciting aspects of dermatology is the ability of the trained eye to observe a cutaneous sign and diagnose a systemic disease – this is one such case. The cutaneous findings of pretibial myxoedema (thyroid dermopathy) point to an underlying thyroid disorder most commonly that of autoimmune Graves's thyrotoxicosis. Pretibial myxoedema may also be seen in Hashimoto's thyroiditis, and primary hypo-/euthyroidism. The exact pathogenesis of the skin changes is yet to be delineated, however it is thought that through an antibody-mediated process skin fibroblasts are stimulated to produce excessive quantities of glycosaminoglycans, which leads to deposition of hyaluronic acid in the skin.

Classically, the development of pretibial myxoedema is insidious with the development of non-pitting oedema over the anterior and lateral shins. Chronic oedema leads to firm indurated pigmented plaque-like areas which may become slightly tender. Skin changes usually follow eye disease and the diagnosis of thyroid disease, however skin changes may be the first sign. Many patients with pretibial myxoedema have thyroid eye disease with proptosis, lid retraction and periorbital oedema. Thyroid acropachy (clubbing) is common in patients with pretibial myxoedema, and onycholysis of the 4th and 5th fingernails may also occur.

Investigations should include thyroid function tests, which usually show very high levels of free thyroxins T4 and T3, and low levels of thyroid-stimulating hormone. Thyrotropin receptor and antithyroglobulin antibodies are usually positive. Skin biopsy is not usually recommended, as healing of the biopsy site may be poor leading to chronic ulceration.

Treatment of pretibial myxoedema is unsatisfactory. Topical or intra-lesional corticosteroids and compression stockings can help to improve the appearance, lessen discomfort and prevent possible ulceration. Trials of intra-lesional octreotide have had mixed success at reducing the levels of hyaluronic acid in the affected skin. Surgery should be avoided as healing is usually poor.

Radioactive iodine is still considered the first-line treatment for Graves's disease with subsequent thyroid replacement necessary in a proportion of patients commencing approximately two months following thyroid gland destruction. For severe Graves's disease ophthalmopathy, high-dose corticosteroids may be required or even orbital decompression surgery.

 KEY POINTS

- Pretibial myxoedema occurs in about 15 per cent of patients with underlying thyrotoxic Graves's disease.
- Deposition of hyaluronic acid in the skin leads to oedematous plaques of the shins.
- Pretibial myxoedema is difficult to manage, however compression and topical steroids may help.

History

A 56-year-old man presents to the dermatology out-patient clinic with a 2-year history of an asymptomatic eruption on his limbs. Lesions initially appeared on the dorsi of his hands, but over the past two years they have also appeared on his elbows and ankles. He is otherwise well.

Examination

He has an erythematous eruption consisting of grouped lesions on his hands, elbows and ankles. On the dorsi of his hands the lesions consist of discrete annular and polycyclic lesions with a raised erythematous edge and central clearing (Fig. 46.1). On palpation the lesions are indurated (firm thickening of the dermis) with no surface change such as xerosis or scaling (normal epidermis).

 INVESTIGATIONS

A skin biopsy was taken. Serum glucose was determined.

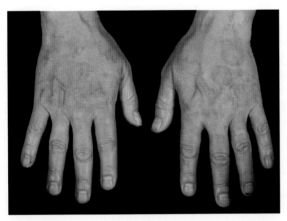

Figure 46.1

Questions

- What is the diagnosis?
- What is the underlying pathophysiology?
- What are the options for treatment?

This man has a cutaneous eruption consistent with the diagnosis of granuloma annulare (GA). This is a relatively common skin eruption that can occur at any age. The asymptomatic lesions characteristically appear symmetrically on the dorsi of the hands and feet and over the flexor surfaces of the wrists and ankles. The onset of the lesions is usually insidious.

The morphology of GA is variable but characteristically there are multiple, grouped, small-diameter, annular erythematous lesions with a raised discrete edge. The centre of the lesions is usually mildly hyperpigmented compared with the surrounding normal skin. Papules, nodules and plaques may also be seen. The skin lesions feel firm on palpation. Disseminated GA is a rare variant of the disease characterized by multiple papules on the trunk and limbs.

There is an increased incidence of GA in association with type 1 diabetes; therefore, testing of fasting blood glucose may be indicated if patients have any systemic symptoms.

The cause of GA remains unknown. Histopathology from affected skin is characterized by areas of degenerative collagen fibres surrounded by palisading granulomas and reactive giant cells. A granulomatous pathology has led to speculation of an infective aetiology.

Treatment of GA is often unsatisfactory, however the eruption can resolve spontaneously. Lesions can demonstrate a reverse Koebner's phenomenon, whereby they resolve following damage though a skin biopsy or cryotherapy. Superpotent topical steroids with/without occlusion for a few weeks may help lesions to disappear more quickly. For problematic lesions over joints intra-lesional triamcinolone can be helpful. There are numerous case reports of other successful treatments including psoralen–UVA, photodynamic therapy, antibiotics, oral prednisolone and ciclosporin.

 KEY POINTS

- Granuloma annulare is an asymptomatic eruption of unknown aetiology.
- Lesions are grouped characteristically over the dorsi of the hands and feet.
- The eruption usually resolves spontaneously, however treatment can be attempted to speed resolution.

History

A 34-year-old man presents to the dermatology clinic with multiple skin lesions on his limbs, which are asymptomatic and have increased in number over one year. He is otherwise well. On direct questioning he admits to shortness of breath whilst playing football.

Examination

He has multiple papules, nodules and annular lesions that are mainly scattered over his limbs (Fig. 47.1). These range in colour from tan/brown to purple. The skin overlying the lesions is slightly shiny and taut. On palpation of the lesions there is neither surface scale or textural change at the surface (epidermis normal), however there is marked induration (a firmness felt in the underlying tissue) indicating dermal pathology. The lesions are non-tender and skin temperature was normal. His temperature is 37 °C, blood pressure 124/87 mmHg, pulse 72 /min and oxygen saturation on air is 96%.

🔍 INVESTIGATIONS

		Normal
C-reactive protein	< 5 mg/L	< 5.0mg/L
Erythrocyte sedimentation rate	21 mm/h	1–10 mm/h
Calcium	2.72 mmol/L	2.15–2.60 mmol/L
Corrected calcium	2.68 mmol/L	2.15–2.60 mmol/L
Angiotensin converting enzyme	103 IU/L	8-52 IU/L

The full blood count was normal.

Kidney and liver function tests were normal

Chest X-ray: Bilateral hilar lymphadenopathy with fibrotic changes in the lower zones

Lung function tests: Mild airflow obstruction, no significant response seen post-bronchodilator

Histopathology from a skin biopsy showed a normal epidermis and multiple, well-formed, non-caseating 'naked' epithelioid granulomas.

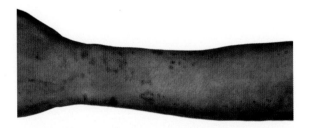

Figure 47.1

Questions

- What tests would you request to help confirm your diagnosis?
- What is your approach to this patient's management?

This man has cutaneous and respiratory sarcoidosis. Skin lesions are classically asymptomatic and firm to touch. The involved skin is usually brown or slightly purplish in colour. Papules, nodules, plaques and annular lesions are often seen. However, some patients may present with just a few flesh-coloured nodules on the face, or purple infiltrated nasal skin (lupus pernio). Some patients may have signs of erythema nodosum (tender nodules on the anterior shins), which results from an underlying panniculitis (inflammation of fat). Approximately 30 per cent of patients with sarcoidosis have cutaneous involvement.

Patients may have palpable lymphadenopathy or evidence of 'bulky hilar' on their chest X-ray. Formal lung function tests should be conducted in patients with respiratory symptoms and/or an abnormal chest X-ray. A skin biopsy from involved skin should be performed to help confirm the diagnosis. The histology classically demonstrates non-caseating 'naked granulomas' within the dermis. The aetiology of sarcoidosis is unknown but is hypothesized to be caused by a persistent antigen of mild virulence leading to chronic T-cell activation and granuloma formation.

Sarcoidosis is frequently managed by a multidisciplinary team, according to which organs are affected. If patients have solely cutaneous involvement, then lesions can be managed with superpotent topical or intra-lesional steroids, oral prednisolone, hydroxy-chloroquine or low-dose methotrexate.

This patient has significant respiratory as well as cutaneous involvement of his sarcoidosis, therefore a systemic approach to his management is indicated. A short course of tapering oral prednisolone (20–40 mg daily) may be commenced initially before switching to steroid-sparing low-dose methotrexate weekly for disease control.

 KEY POINTS

- Cutaneous sarcoid can have a very heterogeneous appearance.
- Cutaneous lesions may signify underlying systemic disease, so always order a systems review.
- In multisystem disease the skin is often the most accessible organ for a histological diagnosis.

History

A 73-year-old retired dinner lady presents with a 4-week history of a non-healing area on her right leg following trauma from a shopping trolley. She tells you that she has 'suffered from her legs' for many years now, complaining of long-standing swelling, aching and itching of her lower legs, particularly towards the end of the day. She is a non-smoker. She has six children. She mentions that her own mother had leg ulcers which never healed. Her only medication is bendroflumethiazide 2.5 mg/day.

Examination

She is overweight (height 1.55 m, weight 78 kg), her blood pressure is 130/70 mmHg, and urine dipstick is negative. There is an irregularly shaped ulcer over the medial malleolus on the right leg (Fig. 48.1). It measures 6.5 × 4 cm at maximum diameter. The surface of the ulcer has some clean adherent slough and the base shows evidence of granulation tissue, the edges of the ulcer are sloping. The surrounding skin is red-brown colour, it is noticeably shiny and feels tight. Her dorsalis pedis pulses are easily palpable bilaterally. The remainder of her examination is unremarkable.

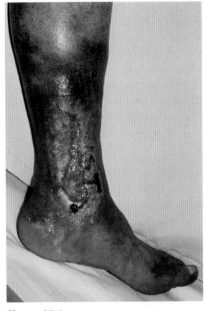

Figure 48.1

Questions

- What is the diagnosis?
- What risk factors does the patient have for this condition?
- How should she be investigated and managed?

ANSWER 48

This clinical presentation would fit best with venous ulcer disease. Venous ulcers are classically found in the gaiter area and may, as in this case, occur on the background of chronic venous dermatitis with consequent lipodermatosclerosis. Lipodermatosclerosis refers to the fibrosis of subcutaneous adipose tissues and is usually accompanied by haemosiderin deposition, erythema, pruritus and trophic changes of the skin. Its presence further impairs wound healing. There may be varicosities and oedema. Preceding venous hypertension may be associated with rather non-specific symptoms.

! Risk factors for venous ulcer disease
• Advancing age
• Male sex (male to female ratio 1.5–10 : 1)
• History of deep vein thrombosis
• History of phlebitis
• Trauma to legs
• Congestive cardiac failure
• Family history of venous ulcers
• Obesity
• Higher number of pregnancies
• Occupation involving prolonged standing

In general the diagnosis of venous ulcer disease is a clinical one based on clinical findings and demonstration of adequate pedal pulses to rule out an element of arterial insufficiency. Where secondary infection is suspected, microbiology swabs should be obtained. A recent expert consensus paper suggests that all patients with venous ulcer should undergo duplex ultrasonography to confirm or exclude venous dysfunction and identify whether the problem is caused by anatomical obstruction, reflux, or both. It is also standard practice to document ankle/brachial index prior to application of compression.

The goals of management are to control symptoms, promote healing and prevent recurrence. A non-surgical approach remains the primary treatment. Bed-rest and elevation is effective but for most impractical, and compression is the 'gold standard'. Compression garments or dressings can be painful and are frequently itchy. The mean time to ulcer healing, even with strict adherence to treatment, is in excess of five months. Surgical intervention to address perforator vein incompetence does not seem to alter outcome but may help to prevent recurrence; there is no effective surgical intervention to address deep venous insufficiency. There are no drugs that promote healing and, in particular, routine use of systemic antibiotics is not indicated.

KEY POINTS

- Venous disease is the most common cause of leg ulcers.
- Symptoms of venous hypertension include aching, a sense of swelling or heaviness, cramps, itch, tingling and restlessness, often worse at the end of the day or after prolonged standing.
- In addition to ulceration at the gaiter area, signs of venous hypertension include varicosities, broken reticulate capillaries, oedema, hyperpigmentation associated with haemosiderin deposition, erythema, loss of hair, or thickened trophic nail changes and ultimately lipodermatosclerosis.

History

A 33-year-old woman attends the dermatology clinic with a 9-month history of unilateral leg swelling. Although the swelling is a cause of significant cosmetic concern, it is fairly asymptomatic. She is otherwise fit and well. She has travelled within France, Sweden and North America over the last 10 years but never visited the tropics. She is not taking any medication. There is no family history of similar swelling or varicose veins.

Examination

There is unilateral swelling of the entire left leg, including toes and extending to the groin. There is no involvement of the skin above the inguinal ligament. The oedema is non-pitting and non-tender. Over the distal anterior shin, the skin is erythematous, with evidence of early verrucous or cobble-stone change (Fig. 49.1), but there is no crusting, oozing or ulceration. There are no palpable lymph nodes. Examination of her cardiorespiratory system, abdomen and pelvis was normal.

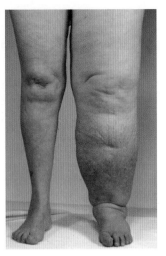

Figure 49.1

INVESTIGATIONS		
		Normal
Haemoglobin	14.9 g/dL	13.3–17.7 g/dL
Mean corpuscular volume	85 fL	80–99 fL
White cell count	6.3×10^9/L	$3.9–10.6 \times 10^9$/L
Platelets	220×10^9/L	$150–440 \times 10^9$/L
Sodium	138 mmol/L	135–145 mmol/L
Potassium	4.2 mmol/L	3.5–5.0 mmol/L
Urea	5.8 mmol/L	2.5–6.7 mmol/L
Creatinine	118 µmol/L	70–120 µmol/L
Albumin	42 g/L	35–50 g/L
Glucose	5.5 mmol/L	4.0–6.0 mmol/L
Bilirubin	15 µmol/L	3–17 µmol/L
Alanine transaminase	33 IU/L	5–35 IU/L
Alkaline phosphatase	188 IU/L	30–300 IU/L
Erythrocyte sedimentation rate	7 mm/h	< 10 mm/h
C-reactive protein	4 mg/L	< 5 mg/L
Urinalysis	Negative for blood, protein and leucocytes	

Questions
- What is the diagnosis?
- What are the potential causes?
- How would you investigate this patient further?

The diagnosis in this patient is unilateral lymphoedema. Differential diagnoses would include deep venous thrombosis (DVT) (although one would anticipate more symptoms and a degree of pitting were that the case) and lipoedema (usually painful and symmetrically bilateral, rarely involving the feet or ankles, but occurring in young adult females).

Lymphatics are essential for clearing extravascular fluid and debris and for the transport of immunocompetent cells during the initiation of an immune response. Lymphoedema is an accumulation of protein-rich (1-5.5 g/mL) interstitial fluid due to impaired functioning of the lymphatic channels. This high protein concentration favours the accumulation of water within the interstitium. This protein and fluid accumulation initiates a marked inflammatory reaction. Macrophage activity is increased, resulting in destruction of elastic fibers and production of fibrosclerotic tissue. Fibroblasts migrate into the interstitium and deposit collagen. The result of this inflammatory reaction is a change from the initial pitting oedema to the brawny non-pitting oedema that is characteristic of lymphoedema. Consequently, local immunologic surveillance is suppressed, and chronic infections, as well as malignant degeneration to lymphangiosarcoma, may occur.

Lymphoedema can be primary or secondary. The primary causes are abnormalities in the lymphatic system that are present at birth, although not always clinically evident until later in life. The causes of secondary lymphoedema include (1) infections, such as recurrent lymphangitis or cellulitis, or worldwide the most common cause, filariasis (the direct infestation of lymph nodes by the parasite *Wuchereria bancrofti*), (2) malignancy, (3) obesity, and (4) scarring following trauma or surgery.

Further investigations should be undertaken to rule out occult malignancy and underlying infection (such as full blood count, CRP and ESR, renal and liver function, tumour markers, abdominal and pelvic imaging studies). Lymphoscintigraphy can be used to assess the lymphatic system: it allows for detailed visualization of the lymphatic channels with minimal risk. The anatomy and the obstructed areas of lymphatic flow can be assessed. Ultrasonography can be used to evaluate the lymphatic and venous systems. Volumetric and structural changes are identified within the lymphatic system. Venous abnormalities such as DVT can be excluded based on ultrasonography findings. Lymphangiography, although once considered the 'gold standard' investigation of lymphatic obstruction, is now rarely performed because of potential adverse effects.

In this case no evidence of occult malignancy was detected on physical examination or following bloods tests and imaging studies. The diagnosis therefore would be of a primary lymphoedema.

Primary lymphoedema has been subdivided into three entities: congenital lymphoedema, lymphoedema praecox, and lymphoedema tarda, depending on age at presentation. These conditions may be sporadic, with no family history, and usually involve the lower extremity almost exclusively. All are thought to result from a (usually localized) developmental abnormality of the lymphatic system, which may only become apparent after a triggering event in later life. Overall women are more commonly affected than men.

The management of lymphoedema is lifelong and is often onerous for the patient; it requires a high degree of compliance to prevent long-term complications. The principles of treatment are to eliminate protein stagnation and restore normal lymphatic circulation. Meticulous hygiene is essential as well as the avoidance of trauma, and a pragmatic approach to weight reduction. Long-term prophylactic antimicrobial treatment might be considered for patients with recurrent cellulitis or lymphangitis. A compression garment should be worn during the day with elevation of the affected limb overnight. Intermittent pneumatic pump compression therapy may also be instituted on an out-patient basis or in the home.

Complications and treatment of lymphoedema

Complications
- Functional effects of swelling – fatigue, embarrassment, difficulty with clothing
- Inflammatory effect of accumulated protein-rich fluid, leading to dermatitis
- Increased infection risk – recurrent fungal (e.g. tinea pedis) and bacterial (e.g. cellulitis, lymphangitis) infections
- Fibrosclerotic changes – leading to woody thickening and peau d'orange appearance and verrucous hyperkeratosis
- Risk of malignant change – lymphangiosarcoma

Treatment
- Fastidious foot-care and skin hygiene
- Consideration of prophylactic antibiotics
- Compression garments and regular appropriate exercise
- Intermittent pneumatic pump compression

KEY POINTS

- Lymphoedema may be primary or secondary. Secondary lymphoedema can result from lymphatic obstruction due to infections, malignancy, obesity, or scarring following trauma or surgery.
- Prevention of complications is a long-term process.
- Surveillance for infection and malignant transformation is part of the long-term follow-up of affected individuals.

History

You are asked to review a painful skin wound on the right heel of an 82-year-old man who is currently convalescing at a residential care home. He has been a resident of the home following a cerebrovascular accident two months ago and although he is showing signs of neurological recovery his mobility is limited by osteoarthritis of the hips and knees. He had coronary artery bypass grafting 8 years ago. He is an ex-smoker. His medications are aspirin 75 mg, atorvastatin 10 mg, lisinopril 10 mg and nifedipine 20 mg daily, as well as codeine and paracetamol prn for pain relief, and a prescription for prn haloperidol 1.5 mg.

Examination

He is a frail man with limited mobility during the examination. His blood pressure is 120/80 mmHg. He has a left-sided upper motor neurone weakness. He has a well-defined area of ulceration over the medial aspect of his left heel (Fig. 50.1). The ulcer is 'punched out' with a dry necrotic eschar overlying the base, the surrounding skin is erythematous. On examination of the arterial system of his legs, the femoral pulses are present but popliteal, posterior tibial and dorsalis pedis pulses are reduced on the left compared with the right. He has normal sensation in his feet. Ankle/brachial indices are measured and demonstrate an ankle pressure of 60 mmHg on the left and 80 mmHg on the right.

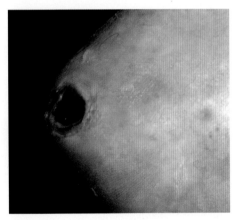

Figure 50.1

Questions

- What is the diagnosis?
- What are the likely factors in the aetiology of this ulcer?
- What is the optimum management?

The diagnosis in this patient is pressure or decubitus ulcer. The ulcer is located over a bony prominence. The history and examination showed that he has arterial disease, and ischaemia leading to tissue necrosis will be an important factor; however an ankle pressure of > 50 mmHg is not considered to represent critical ischaemia. The presence of arterial disease is a poor prognostic feature.

Other contributing factors will be his age and his neurological impairment (particularly the combination of spasticity and paralysis) and reduced mobility due to arthritis. The appropriateness of the prescription for haloperidol should be considered, as excessive sedation will contribute to impaired sensory perception. Other factors to consider are malnutrition, anaemia and incontinence. The aetiology of decubitus ulcers is generally a combination of pressure over bony prominences, shearing forces, destruction of the skin and compromised blood flow.

The prevention and care of chronic lower leg ulceration places a significant burden on patients and the health care system. Non-healing ulcers place the patient at risk for lower extremity amputation. Pressure relief is essential to the management of pressure ulcers using repositioning schedules and specialized beds. Management of incontinence to prevent contamination as well as wound cleaning and appropriate dressing are important to encourage healing and prevent bacterial secondary infection. Necrotic tissue may require surgical debridement. Measures to address immobility and spasticity, nutritional status and lower limb perfusion should be considered.

Staging of pressure ulcers

- Stage I – no tissue loss, non-blanching erythema
- Stage II – superficial, partial-thickness ulcer with skin breakdown and minimal tissue necrosis
- Stage III – full-thickness ulcer displaying breakdown extending through the dermis and exposing subcutaneous tissue
- Stage IV – extends through the deep fascia, damaging underlying muscle and bone

---

 KEY POINTS

- Decubitus ulcers remain a significant cause of morbidity despite advances in their prevention, as well as active medical, surgical and nursing management.
- They particularly affect elderly persons with impaired sensation, prolonged immobility and other complex co-morbidities.
- Recognition and remediation of risk factors and, in particular, pressure relief are crucial to their prevention.

History

A 63-year-old man presents to the dermatology out-patient clinic complaining of a non-healing ulcer on his right foot. He has had poorly controlled type 2 diabetes for 22 years. Four years ago his right big toe was amputated because of ulceration and infection. Following that procedure his compliance with medication improved and he stopped smoking. He attends many different hospital appointments monthly and struggles with his weight because of chronic back pain and impaired vision. His medication includes metformin, glicazide, ramipril, amlodipine, aspirin and simvastatin.

Examination

The patient is 1.85 m tall, weighs 104 kg and his blood pressure is 154/88 mmHg. He has a painless round ulcer overlying the right third metatarsal head, the base of which is covered with purulent slough. The ulcer is surrounded by callus formation with erythema and swelling extending medially and overlying the second metatarsal (Fig. 51.1). There is no tissue crepitus but some scaliness of the surrounding plantar skin. There is onychodystrophy suggestive of onychomycosis affecting four of his nine toenails. He has reduced posterior tibial artery pulses bilaterally and absent dorsalis pedis pulse on the right. Ankle reflexes cannot be elicited. He is unable to sense 10-g monofilament pressure over the medial aspect of the distal third of his right foot; vibration, fine touch and pin-prick sensation are also absent. Furthermore these modalities are reduced at both feet from approximately the ankle level.

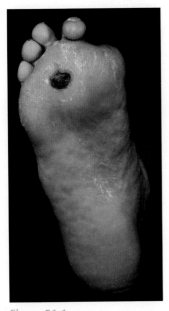

Figure 51.1

		Normal
Haemoglobin	14.4 g/dL	13.3-17.7 g/dL
Mean corpuscular volume	94 fL	80–99 fL
White cell count	9.8×10^9/L	$3.9–10.6 \times 10^9$/L
Platelets	468×10^9/L	$150–440 \times 10^9$/L
Sodium	138 mmol/L	135–145 mmol/L
Potassium	4.8 mmol/L	3.5–5.0 mmol/L
Urea	9.8 mmol/L	2.5–6.7 mmol/L
Creatinine	180 µmol/L	70–120 µmol/L
Albumin	45 g/L	35–50 g/L
Bilirubin	15 µmol/L	3–17 µmol/L
Alanine transaminase	30 IU/L	5–35 IU/L
Alkaline phosphatase	150 IU/L	30–300 IU/L
Erythrocyte sedimentation rate	15 mm/h	< 10 mm/h

Questions

- What factors described in the history and examination contributed to the ulcer?
- Which additional factors described above are risk factors for the development of foot ulceration?
- What additional tests would be performed at the bedside to assess diabetic complications?
- What is the management of this patient's foot ulcer?

Foot ulcers affect 15–25 per cent of patients with diabetes. This patient's peripheral neuropathy is likely to be the direct cause of an ulcer at this site. His elevated blood sugar, peripheral vascular disease and possible ulcer infection contribute to poor healing.

Callus formation often precedes ulceration and in this case reflects abnormal pressure distribution as a result of amputation and neuropathy. Diabetic foot ulcers occur typically over bony prominences of the feet, especially the big toe, or the plantar skin overlying the 1st or 2nd metatarsal heads. Complications of foot ulcers include soft tissue infection (cellulitis, fasciitis) and osteomyelitis. Lower extremity ulcers are a significant factor in amputations amongst diabetics.

Additional bedside tests would include urine dipstick – looking for proteinuria, in particular – and lying and standing blood pressure, as the patient may be describing postural hypotension, a symptom of autonomic neuropathy. A scraping of the scaly areas can be taken to look for tinea pedis and the ulcer should be swabbed for bacterial culture. Blood glucose monitoring may not be informative as it reflects only short-term control. It would, however, be important to check HbA1C level.

The management of diabetic foot ulcers requires modification of factors that contribute to ulcer formation, for example, management of infection and glycaemic control. Standard therapy includes debridement, off-loading and protective dressings. Regular review and inspection of the ulcer is important.

Ulcer prevention is one of the most important interventions medical professionals can provide for diabetic patients. Optimizing glycaemic control and patient education are crucial to ulcer prevention.

Risk factors for the development of foot ulcers in diabetics

- Poor glycaemic control (there is a direct correlation between HbA1C level and incidence of foot ulceration)
- Previous foot ulceration (> 50% will re-ulcerate within 3 years)
- Prior lower limb amputation
- Duration of diabetes (> 10 years)
- Impaired visual acuity (reflecting microvascular disease)
- Onychomycosis

KEY POINTS

- Diabetic ulcers occur over bony prominences often within an area of callus formation.
- Poor glycaemic control, neuropathy and microvascular disease (with or without peripheral vascular disease) are important risk factors.
- Education and support from a multidisciplinary team are important.
- General foot care guidelines for patients with diabetes: daily washing of feet with lukewarm water and careful attention to drying; choice of appropriate footwear (always wear shoes and socks); daily inspection and palpation inside shoes to check for foreign objects or rough surfaces; seeking rapid professional attention for calluses, blisters, cuts, rash or ingrown toe-nails, etc.

History

A 3-year-old girl attends the paediatric dermatology clinic with her mother. She has a red lesion on her left ear, which her mother fears will lead to bullying in school. The lesion is entirely asymptomatic. Her parents first noticed the lesion shortly after birth and describe it as having the appearance of a red 'stain'. Shortly before her six-week check it was beginning to enlarge and it grew until she was approximately four months old. Her mother feels it has been fairly static subsequently. The child is otherwise well; she was born at term and is fully vaccinated to date. There is no family history of birthmarks or other skin lesions.

Examination

She is thriving with height and weight between the 50th and 75th centiles for her age. She has an elevated, dome-shaped, dusky red, rubbery, non-tender lesion on the dorsal aspect of the lobule of her left ear (Fig. 52.1). The overlying skin is showing some patchy pallor (or greying). She has no other skin lesions.

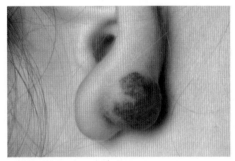

Figure 52.1

Questions

- What is this lesion?
- What is its natural history?
- What management options are available?

This lesion is an infantile haemangioma, also referred to as a capillary haemangioma, strawberry naevus or cavernous haemangioma. These are benign vascular neoplasms and are the most common tumours of infancy. Most infantile haemangiomas are medically insignificant and the vast majority of lesions (80 per cent) are focal and solitary. Occasionally, however, they can impinge on vital structures, ulcerate, bleed, become secondarily infected or painful; also they can cause high-output cardiac failure or significant structural abnormalities or disfigurement. Visual obstruction, airway obstruction or interference with feeding/defaecation are the most commonly encountered complications. Haemangiomas can also occur in extracutaneous sites such as larynx, gastrointestinal tract and other abdominal viscera. Rarely, they may be associated with more extensive underlying congenital anomalies (e.g. PHACE syndrome, posterior fossa brain abnormalities, haemangiomas, arterial lesions, cardiac anomalies and eye abnormalities).

Infantile haemangiomas follow a characteristic course, with an early rapid-proliferation phase during the neonatal period or early infancy, followed by a slow gradual involution phase up to the age of approximately 10 years. Early features include blanching of the affected skin, fine telangiectases, or a red macule or papule. As they proliferate, depending on their size and depth, their appearance may combine one or more features such as dome-shaped, lobulated, plaque-like, and tumoural. Most reach a maximum size of about 5 cm, but they can range from a pin-head to more than 20 cm in diameter. During the involution phase it is common for the haemangioma to shrink centrifugally from the centre; they become less red and gradually duskier (greying) before becoming softer and regaining flesh tones. The involution phase will be completed by 9 years of age in the overwhelming majority of patients, and for approximately 70 per cent of patients the haemangioma resolves completely. In the remainder there may be some residual permanent changes such as telangiectasia, superficial dilated vessels, stippled scarring, epidermal atrophy, hypopigmentation and/or redundant skin with fibrofatty residua.

The majority of infantile haemangiomas, such as the case presented, do not require any medical or surgical intervention. Treatment is indicated to reduce morbidity and mortality and to prevent complications which may have an impact on growth and development. In general the cosmetic aspect of haemangiomas is dealt with following the involution phase. Laser therapy is beneficial in treating ulcerated haemangiomas and thin superficial lesions in cosmetically sensitive sites. Surgical excision is exceptionally rare because of the potential intra-operative hazards and longer-term cosmetic results. Medical treatment with systemic or intra-lesional corticosteroids can be effective at slowing the growth and decreasing the size of proliferating haemangiomas. Propranolol is also emerging as a potentially more effective therapy during the proliferation phase, and has been in use for the management of severe or disfiguring haemangiomas since 2008. Duration of therapy varies from 2 to 10 months and there are currently no universally accepted criteria for initiation of therapy or therapeutic protocols. Propranolol, however, is very likely to make the use of agents such as interferon-α and vincristine obsolete in the management of haemangiomas.

In the case presented it is essential to educate the parents about the natural history and prognosis of infantile haemangiomas, as well as the potential risks and benefits of different treatments. Emotional support and exchange of views are available through forums such as the Birthmark Society. However, there would be little indication for intervention at this stage.

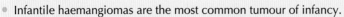

- Infantile haemangiomas are the most common tumour of infancy.
- These benign endothelial neoplasms are typically absent at birth, they characteristically grow rapidly in infancy and gradually spontaneously involute over the first decade.
- The majority of haemangiomas require no treatment; however, if there are associated complications such as visual or airway obstruction, ulceration or bleeding, different treatments are available under close hospital supervision.

History

A 7-week-old baby boy attends the paediatric dermatology clinic with his mother for follow-up of an extensive red patch. He was born at 38 weeks by elective caesarean section for transverse-lie, following an uneventful pregnancy. He has one sister. There is no family history of similar skin lesions. The red patch was noted at birth, and he was reviewed on a daily basis both by the dermatology department and by the neonatal team. No other problems presented prior to discharge on day 5. In particular, his height and weight were both on the 50th centile, he was feeding well, passing urine and meconium. A full blood count was performed prior to discharge and was normal, as was an ultrasound scan of his abdomen, pelvis, spine and head. Since discharge he has continued to thrive, feeding from both breast and bottle. His mother has had contact with health visitors and dermatology specialist nurses and despite considerable initial anxiety is now calm and feels she is coping well.

Examination

His weight is now between the 50th and 75th centiles, with height and head circumference remaining on the 50th centile. He has an extensive, flat (macular), well-defined dusky red patch, which extends from the sole of his left foot along the posterolateral aspect of his leg to involve his entire left buttock and lumbosacral region (Fig. 53.1). He has a similar discrete patch on the left side of his upper abdomen, which extends posteriorly to the midline. Additionally he has a blue-grey macule over his right lumbosacral area (a Mongolian blue spot). His observations are stable and examination of his cardiovascular, respiratory, abdominal systems and genitalia was normal. A detailed neurological examination revealed no concerns, his anterior fontanelle is level and he has a social smile. There is symmetry of all limbs.

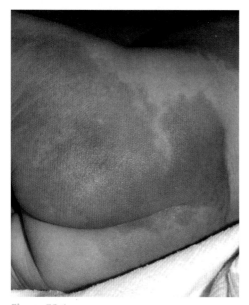

Figure 53.1

		Normal
Haemoglobin	15.3 g/dL	13.3–17.7 g/dL
White cell count	4.3 × 10⁹/L	3.9–10.6 × 10⁹/L
Platelets	225 × 10⁹/L	150–440 × 10⁹/L
Neonatal screening tests	Normal	
Ultrasound scan of abdomen pelvis and head	No evidence of abnormal pelvic, intra-abdominal or intracranial vasculature. No structural abnormalities were detected or evidence of spinal dysraphism	

Questions
- What are these patches?
- What complications can be associated with them?
- How should this child and his family be managed?

These lesions are capillary malformations or port wine stains. They represent congenital malformation of superficial dermal blood vessels as a result of abnormal morphogenesis. In the past, the nomenclature of these lesions has led to confusion and difficulty in differentiating vascular malformations from vascular proliferative lesions such as infantile haemangiomas. Capillary malformations are almost always present at birth (although not always detected because of neonatal plethora) and grow with the child; they remain present for life but may show tendency to colour change (either fading or more commonly becoming a deeper purple). The surface can develop a cobblestone contour or nodularity in adulthood.

Thorough assessment of patients with capillary malformations for associated complications is important. Capillary malformations can occur with other vascular malformations (venous, lymphatic, arterial or mixed). Ocular and/or central nervous system involvement occurs in approximately 10 per cent of patients with facial capillary malformations. In particular, involvement of the distribution of the ophthalmic division of the trigeminal nerve is associated with leptomeningeal involvement (Sturge–Weber syndrome), with risk of glaucoma, seizures, developmental defects, subdural haemorrhages and hemiplegia. All patients with upper facial capillary malformations should have ophthalmological assessment (and magnetic resonance imaging of the brain if Sturge–Weber syndrome is suspected). Klippel–Trenaunay syndrome (angio-osteohypertrophy syndrome) is a triad of capillary malformation, congenital venous malformation and hypertrophy of the underlying tissues including muscle and bone. A capillary malformation overlying the spine may be associated with vascular malformations in the subjacent spinal meninges or occult spinal dysraphism. The coexistence of the capillary malformation and Mongolian blue spot in this case may be coincidental, however the literature suggests the risk of spinal structural or vascular anomalies is higher in the presence of another lumbosacral cutaneous anomaly.

Isolated capillary malformations are not associated with significant medical complications; however, psychosocial disability secondary to disfigurement can be overwhelming. In the neonatal period such obvious and visible differences will inevitably be a source of anxiety for parents and it is crucial that the parents of this baby are offered sympathetic explanations, education and reassurance as well as the opportunity for them to discuss their concerns. They may benefit from peer support through patient support networks.

This child will require long-term follow-up; if associated complications such as limb length discrepancy arise, he will benefit from the care of a multidisciplinary team including dermatology, orthopaedics, interventional radiology, plastic surgery, as well as occupational therapy, physiotherapy, and psychology. The treatment of choice for capillary malformations is pulsed-dye laser, which causes selective destruction of superficial abnormally dilated dermal bloods vessels, by inducing coagulation and rupture. The cosmetic outcome is variable, with larger lesions over limbs responding less well and tending to recur, compared to smaller lesions over the head and neck.

 KEY POINTS

- Capillary malformations are congenital malformations of superficial dermal vessels, which are present at birth and grow with the child.
- They can be associated with other vascular malformations or structural anomalies.
- Isolated capillary malformations can be a source of significant psychosocial morbidity for new parents as well as for the affected individual.

History

A 74-year-old woman presents with a 1-year history of a lesion on the dorsum of her middle finger. This has gradually increased in size over the last 12 months and is asymptomatic. Previously she had a similar lesion on her left leg, which had been treated successfully 18 months ago. She lived abroad as a child and is a keen gardener. She is otherwise well and takes 75 mg aspirin daily.

Examination

There is an erythematous plaque 1 cm in size with overlying scale on the dorsum of her middle finger, the surrounding skin being normal (Fig. 54.1).

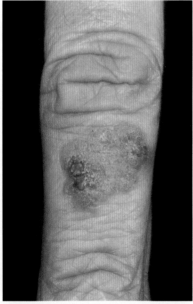

Figure 54.1

Questions

- What are the differential diagnoses?
- How would you confirm the diagnosis?
- What are the options for treatment?

This elderly patient has had significant sun exposure in childhood and now enjoys outdoor activities. The lesion is on a sun-exposed site and has grown slowly. The diagnosis is Bowen's disease – squamous cell carcinoma (SCC) *in situ*. She has had a similar lesion previously. The history of a solitary erythematous plaque with overlying scale on the dorsum of the finger led to a suspicion of Bowen's disease, which was confirmed by taking a biopsy for histopathological analysis.

Bowen's disease appears as a sharply, demarcated, erythematous, patch or plaque with overlying hyperkeratosis. These lesions occur most commonly on the legs of older woman, but also occur on other sun-exposed sites such as the face, ears and the dorsi of the hands. Bowen's disease is a pre-malignant condition, hence the term SCC *in situ*. A SCC is a cancer derived from squamous cells. These are cells that make up the epidermis. *In situ* means that the malignant cells are confined to the epidermis and have therefore not invaded deeper. A change in the appearance of Bowen's disease such as development of a nodule can indicate progression into an invasive SCC.

Bowen's disease occurs in aging skin. It may be caused by ultraviolet irradiation or human papillomavirus (HPV) infection. HPV-induced Bowen's disease occurs mostly in the genital sites but may also appear periungally.

Differential diagnoses include discoid eczema, psoriasis, viral warts, seborrhoeic keratoses, actinic keratoses, superficial basal cell carcinoma and extramammary Paget's disease.

Histolopathology shows full-thickness change of the epidermis with loss of the normal maturation keratinocytes.

Treatments include topical chemotherapy with 5-fluorouracil cream and imiquimod. Cryotherapy with liquid nitrogen is very effective. Photodynamic therapy (PDT) refers to treatment with a photosensitizer that is applied topically to the affected area prior to exposing it to a strong source of visible light. Other destructive methods include curettage and cautery.

 KEY POINTS

- Bowen's disease occurs on sun-exposed skin sites in the elderly.
- Patches are well demarcated, erythematous and hyperkeratotic.
- Bowen's disease is squamous cell carcinoma *in situ*.

History

A 59-year-old construction worker presents to the dermatology clinic with a 3-year history of a slow-growing lesion on the left temple. The patient describes that the lesion had begun as a small 'spot', which had gradually enlarged and had more recently been crusting over and intermittently bleeding. There is no previous history of skin disease and no family history of similar problems. He has worked outdoors for 40 years and has travelled abroad to tropical climates twice a year.

Examination

There is a nodular lesion 18 mm in diameter with a translucent edge and overlying telangiectasia with central crust (Fig. 55.1). Full skin examination does not reveal any other similar lesions, although he is noted as being tanned.

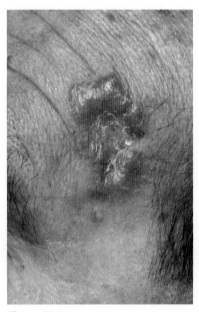

Figure 55.1

Questions

- What is the clinical diagnosis?
- What investigation should be performed?
- How should this patient be treated?

Clinically, this man has a basal cell carcinoma (BCC) or rodent ulcer. Malignant skin tumours are amongst the commonest of all cancers. BCCs are the most common of the skin cancer group and their incidence is continuing to rise. Most typically they are found on sun-exposed sites in lighter skinned, middle-aged to elderly individuals, although owing to changes in lifestyle and increasing travel such patients can present as early as in the third decade.

There are different clinical and histological types. This patient has a nodular BCC, which is the most frequently seen and, like this lesion, has well-defined, rolled edges that have a pearly translucent appearance. On closer examination superficial blood vessels (telangiectasia) are often seen. As the BCC enlarges it can ulcerate, hence the patient's description of recent intermittent bleeding and crusting. Eventually the ulceration can cause destruction of the underlying tissue. For example, around the nasal area the cartilage can be destroyed and hence the name 'rodent' ulcer. This patient's outdoor occupation and recreational history of travel to areas of high intensity ultraviolet are important.

To confirm the diagnosis a skin biopsy was performed for histopathological confirmation. Other subtypes include superficial BCCs, where the lesion is much flatter and erythematous, often with an overlying surface scale (Fig. 55.2). Morphoeic BCCs are translucent plaques with an ill-defined edge (Fig. 55.3).

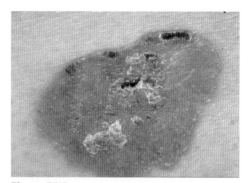

Figure 55.2

Although BCCs have a low malignant potential they are locally destructive and can cause significant morbidity, especially when occurring around facial structures such as the eyes and nose. Treatment is dependent on site, size and type of BCC. Treatment options include curettage and cautery, surgical excision, photodynamic therapy and radiotherapy. For those lesions in high-risk anatomical sites and for lesions that have clinically ill-defined margins, such as the morphoeic BCCs, then Mohs' micrographic surgery is the treatment of choice, where the tissue is sectioned and examined to ensure that all the tumour has been excised before repairing the defect.

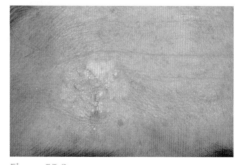

Figure 55.3

Patients should undergo a full skin examination and be given future photoprotective advice.

 KEY POINTS

- Basal cell carcinomas (BCCs) are the most common type of skin cancer.
- Subtypes of BCCs include nodular, superficial and morphoeic.
- Treatment options include curettage and cautery, surgical excision annd radiotherapy.

History

A 36-year-old man presents with multiple skin lesions, which have gradually developed over the last two years. He had been diagnosed with a basal cell carcinoma (BCC) over his left cheek 10 years previously, and this had been removed. He is otherwise well but has undergone numerous dental procedures in the past. His father also had multiple BCCs.

Examination

He has multiple erythematous patches with overlying scale on his anterior and posterior trunk (Fig. 56.1) and three similar lesions on his face. Examination of his hands reveals sharply marginated, depressed lesions 1-2 mm in diameter (Fig. 56.2).

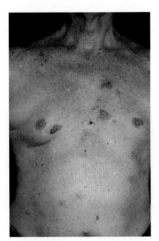

Figure 56.2

Figure 56.1

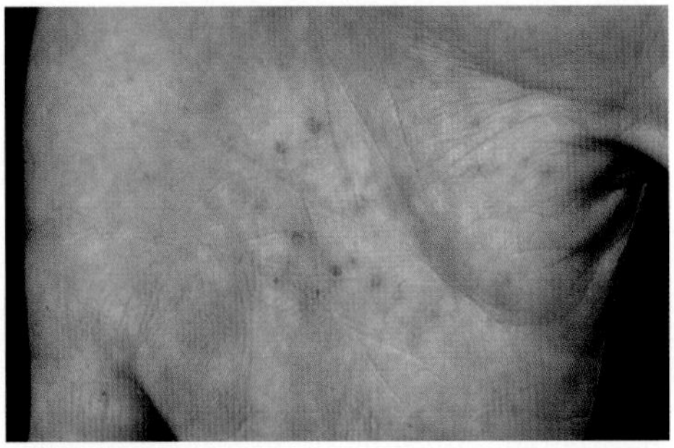

Questions

- What is this syndrome?
- What are the other features?
- How should this patient be managed?

This patient has Gorlin's syndrome (basal cell naevus syndrome). The history of a previous BCC at such an early age combined with now several likely superficial BCCs, which appear as erythematous patches with overlying scale, is highly suggestive of the diagnosis. The palmar pits and family history are also relevant.

Gorlin's syndrome is an autosomal dominant disease caused by a mutation in the patched (PTCH) gene on chromosome 9q (9q22). This gene normally functions as a tumour suppressor, so when defective it allows basal cell carcinomas to develop. It usually presents in late childhood, although some features are congenital.

BCCs can occur from early adolescence and continue throughout life. They are more common on sun-exposed sites, but also occur in unexposed areas and are usually multiple. The most common cutaneous lesions are superficial and nodular BCCs, although morphoeic BCCs can also occur. Small indentations on the palmar surfaces which are pinpoint to several millimeters across are present in 50 per cent of patients. Developmental abnormalities include frontal bossing, odontogenic keratocysts (which was the reason for this patient's dental procedures), bifid or splayed ribs, scoliosis and kyphosis. Eye lesions including strabismus can also occur. Ovarian fibromas and teratomas have also been reported.

Gorlin's syndrome is an important condition to recognize owing to potential development of literally hundreds of BCCs in one lifetime, which leads to multiple excisions and considerable scarring. Patients with suspected Gorlin's syndrome should be referred for genetic counselling. Life-long photoprotection and follow-up is the mainstay of treatment.

Management of superficial BCCs, which are the main type in these patients, includes topical therapy with the immunomodulator imiquimod 5% cream. Destructive methods, such as cryotherapy with liquid nitrogen and curettage and cautery, are effective. Photodynamic therapy (PDT) and surgical excision are also therapeutic options.

 KEY POINTS

- Gorlin's syndrome is an autosomal dominant disease caused by a mutation in the PTCH gene.
- Patients develop multiple BCCs.
- Other manifestations include palmar pits, frontal bossing and jaw cysts.

History

An 86-year-old man presents with a bleeding lesion on his scalp. This had slowly enlarged over a 4-month period and was very painful. He had worked abroad whilst in the army 50–60 years ago. He had previously had other lesions treated on the scalp with liquid nitrogen.

Examination

There is a large ulcerated eroded nodule over the vertex of the scalp that is friable, erythematous and with a soft fleshy margin (Fig. 57.1). Over the surrounding skin there are scattered erythematous patches with overlying scale. There is palpable lymphadenopathy in the cervical chain.

 INVESTIGATIONS

A skin biopsy was performed.

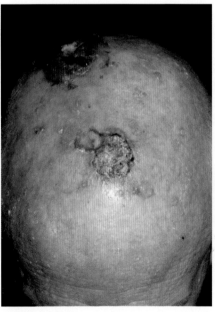

Figure 57.1

Questions

- What is the likely diagnosis?
- How should this patient be treated?

The likely diagnosis is an invasive squamous cell carcinoma (SCC). This patient, an elderly man, has a friable lesion on a bald scalp, which has developed over four months. Initially, SCCs begin as ill-defined, erythematous papules or nodules with a hyperkeratotic top (rough surface); as they enlarge they may ulcerate. He had worked in tropical climates whilst in the armed forces. The palpable cervical nodes suggest that the skin cancer may have metastasized.

The differential diagnoses would include an amelanotic malignant melanoma, and a nodular basal cell carcinoma, actinic keratoses, Bowen's disease and a keratoacanthoma. Invasive SCC is a malignant tumour of keratinocytes. SCCs often arise in precancerous lesions in otherwise healthy individuals over the age of 55 years. Men are more commonly affected than women. SCCs usually arise from actinic keratoses and Bowen's disease. Actinic keratoses are single or multiple erythematous patches with adherent scale on sun-exposed skin in middle-aged adults.

Histologically, there are different levels of differentiation, which can correlate to the aggressiveness of the SCC: well, moderately and poorly differentiated. Poorly differentiated lesions do not show signs of keratinization and clinically appear fleshy, friable and ulcerated as in this case. Metastasis is more common than with well-differentiated lesions.

Predisposing factors include chronic actinic damage, sites of chronic ulceration and scarring, exposure to ionizing radiation and immunosuppression, especially in solid organ transplant recipients and HIV disease.

Surgical excision is the treatment of choice. Depending on location and size of the lesion, it may require closure with a skin flap or graft. Mohs' micrographic surgery may be required for difficult sites. In elderly patients, SCCs can be treated with radiotherapy if surgery is not feasible/desirable. SCCs are more aggressive than basal cell carcinomas and can metastasize. The majority of ultraviolet-induced lesions have a low rate of distant metastasis. Higher risk SCCs are defined as those on the ear, lip and genitalia. A greater incidence of metastases occurs in immunosuppressed patients. All patients with SCCs should have a full skin check to exclude any further suspicious lesions and all lymph node groups examined to exclude metastases. Suspicious nodes should be biopsied.

 KEY POINTS

- Invasive squamous cell carcinoma (SCC) is a malignant tumour of keratinocytes.
- SCCs usually arise from actinic keratoses and Bowen's disease.
- Metastases can spread into the draining lymph nodes and ultimately the blood.

History

A 59-year-old man presents with a 7-week history of a rapidly growing lesion on the dorsum of his right hand. He had seen his GP who had referred him to the dermatology out-patient clinic. However, over the past week the patient had thought that the lesion was now getting smaller and had wondered about cancelling his appointment. His wife had insisted that he attend the clinic to put her mind at rest. He is otherwise well and denies any previous skin problems.

Examination

He has an erythematous, firm, dome-shaped nodule measuring 1.3 cm in diameter with a central keratin plug (Fig. 58.1). Full skin examination reveals a somewhat sun-damaged skin with freckling and solar lentigos but nothing else of note.

 INVESTIGATIONS

A biopsy was arranged.

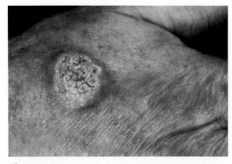

Figure 58.1

Questions

- What is the most likely diagnosis?
- What is the usual course and prognosis of this lesion?

The diagnosis of keratoacanthoma should always be considered when a patient presents with a rapidly enlarging nodule with a central crater. These lesions grow rapidly over a few weeks and are occasionally painful. They typically appear on sun-exposed sites, such as the face and the dorsal surfaces of the hands. Clinically they appear as dome-shaped nodules with shouldering that has a central keratin plug. If the plug falls away a crater is left. Although a keratoacanthoma may mimic a squamous cell carcinoma (SCC) the latter would not spontaneously regress which can occur with keratoacanthomas over a period of weeks to months.

Keratoacanthomas are epidermal tumours, which may behave in a benign way and are therefore called 'pseudo' tumours. In some cases there is a preceding history of minor trauma at the affected site. Previous ultraviolet light exposure appears to be a risk factor, as does human papilloma virus infections. Histologically, they can be difficult to distinguish from SCCs as they contain cytologically atypical keratinocytes. For this reason they can usually only be distinguished on clinical grounds.

SCC is a skin cancer that can metastasize early into the blood. Therefore, most dermatologists would excise such nodules to be sure they have always fully eradicated any potential SCCs. It is not current clinical practice to wait for keratoacanthomas to regress: they are treated as if they were SCCs.

In the right clinical context, where the suspicion of keratoacanthoma is very high and the patient deemed unsuitable for a full excision, some keratoacanthomas may be removed by curettage and cautery (tumour curettage – performed aggressively using three passes) with satisfactory results. If keratoacanthomas involute spontaneously, then they usually leave a cosmetically disfiguring residual scar. Hypertrophic actinic keratoses may also be included in the differential diagnosis.

Finally, a rare genetic disease called Ferguson–Smith syndrome is an autosomal dominant condition where multiple keratoacanthomas develop over the face and extremities. In Ferguson–Smith syndrome the keratoacanthomas do regress spontaneously but lead to significant scarring.

 KEY POINTS

- Keratoacanthomas manifest as dome-shaped nodules with a central keratin plug.
- Histologically they are difficult to distinguish from SCCs.
- Keratoacanthomas may spontaneously regress.

History

A 49-year-old woman presents with a 20-year history of a nodule on her face, which she felt had slowly increased in size over the years. She is anxious about the lesion as friends and neighbours have starting asking her what it is. She feels embarrassed by the lesion and is keen to have it removed. There is no history of itching or bleeding of the lesion. She has quite fair skin (Fitzpatrick type II) and has had limited sun exposure.

Examination

She has a dome-shaped, firm, flesh-coloured nodule lateral to her left eye (Fig. 59.1). There is no surface change felt over the nodule, no telangiectasia and no tenderness. Full skin examination does not reveal any other lesions of note.

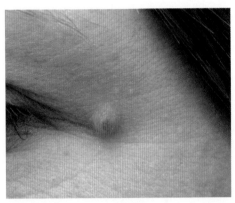

Figure 59.1

Questions

- What is this lesion?
- Can you classify this lesion on clinical grounds?
- How would you manage this patient?

This nodule is a benign intradermal naevus, otherwise known as a 'mole'. A naevus from the word 'nest' is a benign proliferation of cells, as in this case melanocytes. Naevi may be congenital or acquired and may contain melanocytes, epidermal cells or connective tissue.

Melanocytic naevi are very common and are usually multiple. Naevi may be macular or papular/nodular, they vary in colour from pink or flesh-coloured to dark brown or black. Most are round or oval in shape. They are usually < 1 cm in diameter and are common in patients of skin types I–IV and less common in types V and VI.

Melanocytic naevi are classified accordingly to their histology. They are described according to the site of the naevus cells in the skin (Fig. 59.2). The naevus cells in melanocytic naevi are thought to be derived from melanocytes that migrate to the epidermis during embryonic development from the neural crest.

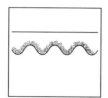 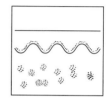

Junctional naevus   Compound naevus   Intradermal naevus

Figure 59.2

Melanocytic naevi begin as a proliferation of cells along the dermo-epidermal junction, forming a junctional naevus. Clinically these moles tend to be flat and dark brown (Fig. 59.3). With continued proliferation, cells extend from the dermo-epidermal junction into the dermis, forming nests of naevus cells, so-called compound naevus. Clinically these moles have a centrally raised area and may be surrounded by flat pigmentation (Fig. 59.4). Finally, the junctional component of the naevus may resolve leaving an intradermal naevus, as in this patient. These moles often protrude from the skin surface and are flesh-coloured or slightly pigmented.

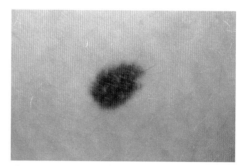

Figure 59.3

Acquired melanocytic naevi appear throughout childhood and adolescence reaching a peak in early adulthood. They may also appear in later adult life, usually secondary to excessive ultraviolet light exposure for the skin type. In the 60th decade onwards naevi usually gradually involute and many disappear altogether.

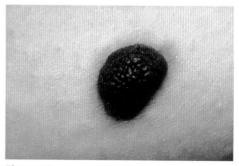

Figure 59.4

This patient should be reassured that her mole is benign. She should be given sun-protection advice as she has fair skin and is liable to get sunburn in strong sunlight.

Acquired moles should be distinguished from congenital melanocytic naevi (CMNs), which are usually present at birth or appear in the first year of life. Approximately 1 per cent of Caucasians are affected. The lesions are usually > 1 cm in diameter and can become protuberant and hairy in nature with increasing age. CMNs usually grow in proportion to the child – sudden increase in growth, satellite lesions appearing at the periphery or nodules forming within them warrant a skin biopsy. The risk of malignant transformation (melanoma) is thought to be very low but is more often reported in so-called 'giant naevi' which are > 20 cm in diameter.

 KEY POINTS

- A naevus is a benign proliferation of melanocytes.
- Naevi can be junctional, compound or intradermal.
- Naevi are either congenital or acquired.

History

A 28-year-old woman presents with multiple naevi, which had gradually appeared over
many years, since puberty. She denies any history of obvious change in her moles but
feels she has had too many to keep a proper check on them. She reports that all her family have multiple naevi. Her brother on a routine check had recently been diagnosed with
a malignant melanoma.

Examination

She has multiple naevi over her trunk and limbs, all of which have a similar appearance,
with a slightly irregular border and varying shades of brown, tan and light red (Fig. 60.1).

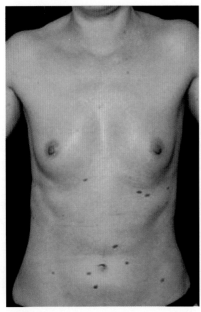

Questions

- What is this syndrome?
- How would you manage this patient?

Figure 60.1

This patient was diagnosed with atypical (dysplastic) naevus syndrome. The patient has multiple atypical naevi, as do her family and a first-degree relative with a malignant melanoma.

Single atypical naevi are present in 5 per cent of the population. These naevi are usually larger than the rest of the patient's moles and clinically have an asymmetrical shape, irregular border and outline. These moles tend to 'stand-out from the crowd'. They have a greater variation in pigmentation than the rest of the patient's moles. These atypical naevi tend to occur later in childhood than common, acquired melanocytic naevi. Histologically these moles show features of mild to severe architectural dysplasia.

Atypical melanocytic naevi occur sporadically or as part of the familial atypical naevus syndrome (patients with this syndrome may have several hundred atypical naevi) and are potential precursors for malignant melanoma.

To be diagnosed with the atypical naevus syndrome patients must have:

1. one or more first-degree or second-degree relatives with malignant melanoma;
2. a large number of naevi (often more than 50), some of which are atypical naevi clinically;
3. histologically dysplastic naevi.

Patients with atypical naevi have a slightly higher risk of developing melanoma than the general population, particularly if they have five or more. Patients with the atypical naevus syndrome have a far greater risk of developing melanoma than those with a small number of atypical moles.

Consequently, patients diagnosed with this syndrome should undergo life-long surveillance due to the potential risk of development of malignant melanoma. Patients are taught to examine their own skin and told what signs to look for, namely, change in size, shape or colour. Photographic and dermatoscopic records are helpful for monitoring these patients to detect early change. Any suspicious or changing atypical naevus should be removed by excision biopsy. Careful photoprotection and sun avoidance are essential.

 KEY POINTS

- Atypical melanocytic naevi occur sporadically or as part of the familial atypical naevus syndrome.
- Patients with this syndrome have a far greater risk of developing melanoma.
- Patients diagnosed with this syndrome should undergo life-long surveillance.

History

A 73-year-old man presents with an 18-month history of a pigmented lesion on his left cheek. He had not paid much attention to it and had assumed it to be a 'sun spot'; however, his daughter is concerned that it has been enlarging slowly and appears to be getting darker in colour. She had taken her father to the GP who had then referred him to the dermatology out-patient department. The patient is a retired roofer and keen gardener. He takes aspirin and an antihypertensive medication.

Examination

The patient has a brown to black macular lesion measuring 2 cm in diameter that has a highly irregular border over his left cheek (Fig. 61.1). He is tanned but otherwise his full skin check is unremarkable.

 INVESTIGATIONS

An incisional skin biopsy was performed.

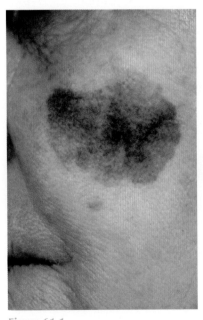

Figure 61.1

Questions

- What is the most likely diagnosis?
- What diagnosis should be excluded?
- How would you manage the patient?

Patients presenting with large pigmented lesions on their skin appearing in later life always warrant referral to a dermatology specialist. This elderly patient had an outdoor occupation before retirement and now spends long hours outside in the garden. Clinically the most likely diagnosis is lentigo maligna (LM). These lesions usually appear in the seventh to eighth decades of life. Sun-exposed sites including the face, neck and dorsi of the hands are most commonly affected. Large macules appear with highly irregular borders and significant variation of pigmentation from tan, brown to black. LM can be a precursor for malignant melanoma *in situ*, so-called lentigo maligna melanoma (LMM). Dermatologists have a low threshold for performing a biopsy from these lesions to exclude malignant transformation. Sampling such large lesions with small punch biopsies, however, may lead to sampling errors and the clinical appearance of the lesion is also important in determining the ultimate management.

Histopathologically, LM is characterized by abnormal melanocytes confined within the epidermis above the basement membrane. When atypical melanocytes invade the rich vascular and lymphatic networks of the dermis, then this becomes LMM.

Possible risk factors for LM include ultraviolet light exposure, fair skin types and occupational risks. Differential diagnoses include solar and seborrhoeic keratoses and LMM.

The definitive treatment of LM is surgical excision. In many patients, however, surgery may not be possible due to other co-morbidities. Other modalities of treatment that may be considered include radiotherapy, cryotherapy and topical imiquimod 5% cream (which is an immunomodulator).

The development of a papular or nodular element within the LM should lead to a high suspicion of transformation to melanoma. LMM makes up 15 per cent of UK malignant melanomas.

 KEY POINTS

- Lentigo maligna (LM) occurs in the seventh or eighth decades on sun-exposed skin.
- LM can be a precursor for malignant melanoma.
- The definitive treatment of LM is surgical excision.

History

A 68-year-old patient presents with a 3-year history of a rash surrounding her right nipple, which is red and mildly pruritic. She denies any discharge from the nipple. Topical steroids prescribed by her GP had been ineffective so she was referred to the dermatology out-patient clinic. The patient has a history of eczema as a child and asthma. More recently she has developed irritation on her hands since looking after her grand daughter 3 days per week. She is otherwise well and takes hormone replacement therapy.

Examination

There is a sharply demarcated erythematous plaque surrounding the right nipple with some slight overlying scale, measuring 6 cm in diameter (Fig. 62.1). There is no obvious underlying breast mass or axillary lymphadenopathy. The left nipple is normal and full skin examination does not reveal any further similar areas. On the dorsi of her hands she has an eczematous rash in the finger webs and under her wedding ring.

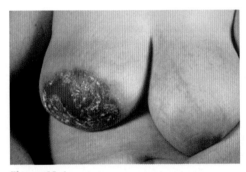

Figure 62.1

Questions

- What is the most likely diagnosis?
- How would you investigate this patient?
- What treatment options are possible?

Asymmetrical 'eczema' of the nipple that is unresponsive to topical steroids should always raise the possibility of an underlying malignancy of the breast. Patients should be referred for consideration of an urgent skin biopsy. This patient was diagnosed with Paget's disease of the right nipple. This represents the intra-epidermal spread of an intraductal breast carcinoma. Although clinically this may mimic eczema a high index of suspicion is needed if the patient is elderly, the disease is asymmetrical and largely unresponsive to conventional eczema therapy. This patient did have a history of atopy; however, atopic eczema of the nipple, although very common, is usually symmetrical and responds rapidly to topical corticosteroids.

Paget's disease is uncommon and involves the nipple or areola, and manifests as erythematous, well-demarcated plaques with overlying scale. It is most commonly seen in woman over 50 years of age. Onset, as in this case, is usually very insidious. Lesions can be asymptomatic or pruritic, painful, oedematous, bleeding or ulcerated. Sometimes nipple retraction and discharge may occur. An underlying breast mass is palpable in less than 50 per cent of patients.

A skin biopsy should be performed from the affected skin. A mammogram and further work-up of any palpable breast mass is vital.

As with any other breast cancer, treatment consists of surgery, radiotherapy and/or chemotherapy. Prognosis is variable and is worse when associated with an underlying breast mass and lymph node involvement.

A similar condition called extramammary Paget's disease may occur away from the nipple and present with a similar eczema-like eruption, usually around the female/male anogenital region or axilla. It is histologically similar to Paget's disease and may be associated with intra-epidermal spread of a ductal apocrine carcinoma of the lower gastrointestinal tract, urinary or female genital tract.

 KEY POINTS

- Paget's disease should be suspected when presented with asymmetrical 'eczema' of the nipple.
- An underlying breast mass is palpable in less than 50 per cent of patients.
- Extramammary disease occurs mainly around the female/male anogenital region.

History

A 39-year-old woman presents to the dermatology 'two-week-wait' clinic with a changing pigmented lesion on her leg. Her partner reported that it had been changing over the last five months. She has type II skin and had moved to the United Kingdom from Australia 5 years previously. Whilst in Australia she had regular skin checks as her father had been diagnosed with malignant melanoma 6 years previously. She is otherwise well and takes no medication other than the oral contraceptive pill.

Examination

She has an asymmetrical, macular, variably pigmented lesion measuring 1.4 cm in diameter on her posterior calf (Fig. 63.1). With the dermatoscope the dermatologist notes a central whitish/blue area in the centre.

 INVESTIGATIONS

Excision of the lesion was performed.

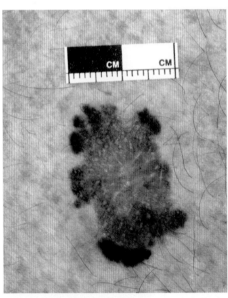

Figure 63.1

Questions

- What is the diagnosis?
- How would you determine the prognosis?
- What management would you organize?

This pigmented lesion looks highly abnormal as it is asymmetrical, has an irregular border and colour and therefore, clinically, is a malignant melanoma. This patient was brought up in Australia where ultraviolet light is intense; a change in the mole had been noted and she had a positive family history of malignant melanoma (MM).

Malignant melanoma is a malignant skin tumour of melanocytes. It is the most aggressive type of skin cancer. Its incidence has doubled in the past decade. Melanoma is amongst the commonest type of cancer in young adults. Approximately 30 per cent of melanomas arise in a pre-existing naevus and the rest appear de novo. MM is more common in Fitzpatrick skin types I and II and has an increasing incidence closer to the equator. The aetiology is complex, however. It is known that genetic predisposition and ultraviolet light exposure (particularly intermittent sun-burning episodes) are likely to play a role.

A pigmented lesion that demonstrates significant change should be excised to exclude melanoma. The A-B-C-D-E rule of melanoma is a useful tool for determining if a lesion is suspicious:

A – Asymmetrical shape
B – Border or Bleeding. The outline of a mole should be regular.
C – Colour. Benign naevi have a uniform colour. Those naevi with differing pigment should be evaluated carefully.
D – Diameter. Melanomas are usually > 6mm in diameter.
E – Evolution: any change noted in a mole

There are four main different variants of melanoma:

- *Superficial spreading melanoma* is the most common type and has a female preponderance. The lower leg is a common site. Clinically, the lesions are usually enlarging brown/black macules with irregular margins and varying degrees of pigmentation. Some lesions may show signs of regression (areas of paleness/whiteness within).
- *Nodular melanoma* is more common in men and is most frequently reported on the posterior trunk. Clinically it appears as a pigmented papule or nodule that may ulcerate. During its horizontal phase of growth, the melanoma is normally flat, that is, superficial spreading melanoma. A nodular melanoma occurs as the vertical phase develops and the melanoma becomes clinically thickened and raised.
- *Acral lentiginous melanomas* occur on the palmar plantar regions and subungal sites. They are the most common form of melanoma in Fitzpatrick skin types IV-VI. Acral melanomas may present as a pigmented macule or as a black area around the subungal skin and nail (Fig. 63.2). The diagnosis is frequently delayed due to the skin sites affected and patients' lack of awareness, hence they often present late with a poor prognosis.
- *Lentigo maligna melanoma* is a melanoma that arises within a lentigo maligna.

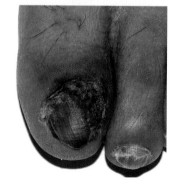

Figure 63.2

 KEY POINTS

- Malignant melanoma (MM) is the most aggressive type of skin cancer.
- It is more common in Fitzpatrick skin types I and II.
- Variants include superficial spreading, nodular, acral and lentigo maligna melanomas.

History

A 29-year-old man presents with a nodule over his posterior trunk. He had recently moved into a flat with friends who had noticed the lesion and advised him to go to the GP. As far as the patient can remember he has had a mole on his back since childhood at the site of the nodule. He has Fitzpatrick skin type I and always burns in the sun, if not careful, and never tans. His family is also fair skinned. He is otherwise well and takes no medication.

Examination

There is a reddish brown nodule arising from a deeply pigmented, irregular macule with variable colour (Fig. 64.1). Full skin examination reveals freckling over his face and shoulders and multiple acquired moles which looked benign.

INVESTIGATIONS

Excision of the lesion was performed.

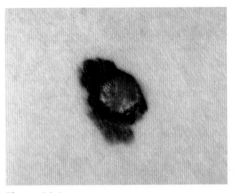

Figure 64.1

Questions
- What is the likely diagnosis?
- What determines his prognosis?
- How should this patient be managed?

This young man has a nodular pigmented lesion on the posterior trunk that has changed in size, shape and colour. The clinical appearance of this lesion should immediately raise the possibility of a nodular malignant melanoma.

Any patient concerned about a mole or skin lesion should have a full skin examination to check all their moles. A suspected melanoma should be excised for histological analysis with a 2-mm margin around it. The pathologist will report the thickness of the melanoma – the Breslow thickness (local invasion) in millimetres. This is the measurement between the granular cell layer to the deepest identifiable melanoma cell. The full skin check of a patient with a suspected malignant melanoma should also include examination of the lymph nodes.

The 'gold standard' treatment of melanomas is surgical. The extent of surgery depends on the thickness of the melanoma and its site. A small area of normal skin around the melanoma is also excised to ensure that all melanoma cells have been removed. This is termed a wide local excision (WLE). For lesions with a Breslow thickness of < 1 mm a 1-cm WLE is required; for lesions > 1 mm a 2-cm WLE is advised. For these thicker melanomas a technique called a sentinel lymph node biopsy may be offered to patients to exclude lymphatic spread. The sentinel lymph node biopsy can predict the presence of clinically non-detectable metastatic melanoma within regional lymph nodes through histopathology. The first node draining a lymphatic basin is termed the 'sentinel node'. If positive, a full basin clearance is offered and all the nodes are examined for further micro-metastases.

If the melanoma has spread to distant sites adjuvant therapies may be offered, but the prognosis is very poor. Distant metastases most commonly occur in lungs, liver, brain, bone and intestines.

Prognosis is determined by the staging classification: local disease T 1–4 a, b; disease in the regional lymph nodes N 1–3; and distant spread M 1a, b, c. The thinner the Breslow thickness, the better the prognosis. For those patients whose melanoma is > 4 mm thick, 50 per cent will die within 5 years.

Following diagnosis, regular follow-up is essential to detect any recurrence. This includes local, lymphatic (lymph nodes) and blood borne (to distant sites). Examination of the scar site to exclude in-transit metastases, full skin examination, lymph node checks and palpation for organomegaly are required. A full systematic review should also be performed to exclude any distant spread. The periodicy and regularity of follow-up is also determined by the stage of the melanoma.

 KEY POINTS

- Patients with a changing naevus should have a full skin examination.
- Breslow thickness measures the invasion depth of a melanoma in millimetres.
- Sentinel lymph node biopsy predicts clinically non-detectable metastatic disease.

History

A 54-year-old woman presents with a widespread eruption that has persisted for almost 20 years. She had initially noticed the first few patches over her pelvic girdle, but slowly over the years the patches have become more widespread. The patches are occasionally mildly itchy; she has noticed a slight dryness over their surface. She has tried over-the-counter antifungal creams and emollients with no real benefit. She is systemically well and takes hormone replacement therapy.

Examination

There is an extensive eruption of multiple erythematous patches with overlying scale over the trunk and limbs, occurring predominantly in unexposed areas (Fig. 65.1). The patches are oval to annular in shape and most, but not all, are well demarcated. Some of the areas are thicker, forming thin plaques.

 INVESTIGATIONS

A skin biopsy was performed.

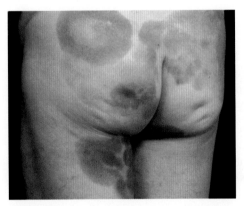

Figure 65.1

Questions

- What is the diagnosis?
- What are the differential diagnoses?
- What are the options for treatment?

Any patient presenting with a very long history of a slowly progressive skin eruption that is unresponsive to topical therapy warrants a skin biopsy. The diagnosis that shouldn't be missed is mycosis fungoides, a form of cutaneous T-cell lymphoma (CTCL). This patient is typical of those presenting with an indolent rash over many years that has a predilection for the pelvic girdle. The condition in the early stages classically presents with erythematous patches with fine overlying scale.

CTCL encompasses 65 per cent of all cutaneous lymphomas. Mycosis fungoides is the commonest of these, accounting for almost half of all cases. It is a low-grade T-cell lymphoma in which there is an abnormal neoplastic proliferation of lymphocytes of a 'T' subtype (thymus-derived). There is a male predominance and it has an incidence of 1 per 100 000 per year.

The average time from disease onset to diagnosis is 7 years. Patients may be misdiagnosed with psoriasis, parapsoriasis, discoid eczema or tinea corporis. Even for an experienced dermatologist the diagnosis may be a challenge, as several skin biopsies may be required to finally clinch the suspected diagnosis of CTCL. Histopathology classically shows atypical lymphocytes in the upper dermis extending into the epidermis with epidermotropism and Pautriers' microabscesses. T-cell gene rearrangement studies from skin biopsies can help to confirm the diagnosis by showing a clone of abnormal T-lymphocytes.

CTCL has three skin stages:

1. *Patch stage:* macular erythema to patches with overlying scale predominantly over non-exposed skin. Spontaneous resolution, fixed lesions and slow progression may be seen. Involved skin can be pruritic and atrophic (thinned).
2. *Plaque stage:* The patches become thickened and form plaques.
3. *Tumour stage:* Large irregular nodules develop within plaques, or de novo. At this stage, spread to other organs is more likely than in the earlier stages.

CTCL may remain confined to the skin for many years running an indolent course, but the abnormal cells can eventually infiltrate other tissues including blood, lymph nodes and visceral sites, usually in the context of extensive cutaneous involvement with widespread plaques, tumours or erythroderma. Unlike some other lymphomas, the prognosis is generally good. However, acurate diagnosis and staging is critical in determining the prognosis of those with CTCL. Investigations therefore are tailored to the clinical setting.

Management of patients should be carried out by a multidisciplinary team. Currently, treatment is not curative but is aimed at controlling symptoms and cosmesis whilst limiting toxicity. Early-stage disease is treated with skin-directed therapy such as topical corticosteroids, phototherapy (psoralen–UVA) and radiotherapy. Patch-stage disease usually improves with topical and phototherapy whereas more infiltrated plaques may require radiotherapy. More advanced disease requires more aggressive treatment including extracorporeal photophoresis, oral retinoids, interferon, single-agent and multi-agent chemotherapy, and even stem-cell bone marrow transplantation.

 KEY POINTS

- Mycosis fungoides is the most common form of cutaneous T-cell lymphoma.
- It is an indolent rash that has a predilection for the pelvic girdle.
- It may infiltrate other tissues including blood, lymph nodes and visceral sites.

History

A 63-year-old man presents to the dermatology out-patient clinic with a slowly growing nodule on his back. He had been unaware of it but his wife is worried as she feels that it has grown over the past year. There is no previous history of skin problems. He takes amlodipine, aspirin and simvastatin and is systemically well.

Examination

There a 3 cm × 3 cm red to plum coloured, firm, non-tender, solitary nodule with a smooth surface on his back (Fig. 66.1). Full skin examination does not reveal any further lesions and there is no evidence of peripheral lymphadenopathy.

 INVESTIGATIONS

A skin biopsy was performed.

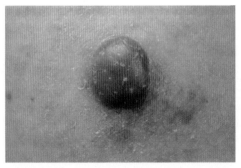

Figure 66.1

Questions

- What are the clinical differential diagnoses?
- How should the patient be managed?
- What is the prognosis?

The differential diagnoses of a firm, indurated erythematous purple papule/nodule that remains fixed for a period of time on the trunk include sarcoid, cutaneous metastasis B-cell lymphoma, Kaposi's sarcoma, and a keloid scar. Skin biopsy with histopathology and immunophenotyping should help to clarify the diagnosis.

This patient was diagnosed with cutaneous B-cell lymphoma, CBCL (a primary cutaneous follicle centre cell lymphoma). CBCL develops when a clonal proliferation of B lymphocytes is confined to the skin. Primary cutaneous lymphomas of the B-cell type comprise approximately 20 per cent of cutaneous lymphomas. Other types of CBCL include primary cutaneous marginal zone, primary cutaneous large B-cell, leg type, and primary cutaneous diffuse large B-cell lymphomas.

Follicle centre cell lymphomas are clinically characterized as asymptomatic nodules, plaques or tumours. CBCL lesions are slow-growing, usually red to plum in colour and are firm with a smooth surface. Common sites include the trunk, scalp and forehead. Primary CBCL needs to be differentiated from a secondary cutaneous lymphoma, which is where a nodal follicular lymphoma has metastasized to involve the skin. This can be differentiated by molecular techniques to demonstrate a lack of the t (14;18) chromosomal translocation.

For solitary lesions or small groups, the treatment of choice is local radiotherapy. For those patients with multiple lesions at distant sites, then chemotherapy may be required. The prognosis is excellent with a 5-year survival of more than 95 per cent.

For the other cutaneous subtypes, patients should be investigated thoroughly for nodal and extracutaneous disease. These investigations include peripheral blood studies, bone marrow biopsy, radiographic imaging and, if indicated, lymph node biopsy.

 KEY POINTS

- Cutaneous B-cell lymphoma (CBCL) occurs when a clonal proliferation of B lymphocytes is confined to the skin.
- Follicle centre cell lymphomas are characterized as asymptomatic nodules.
- Prognosis is excellent with a 5-year survival of more than 95 per cent.

History

A 25-year-old woman presents to the dermatology clinic with a long history of a facial eruption that has been getting worse progressively over the past few years. Some of the lesions on her face are painful at times and sometimes heal with scarring. The rest of her skin is unaffected. Her GP had prescribed several prolonged courses of tetracycline antibiotics with little benefit, and she was unable to tolerate erythromycin due to its gastrointestinal side effects. She took Dianette (oral contraceptive pill) for several months but this had to be stopped as it was significantly lowering her mood.

Examination

There are numerous comedomes, particularly on her forehead, pustules, papules, inflammatory lesions, cysts and atrophic scars (Fig. 67.1). There is sparing of the periorbital skin.

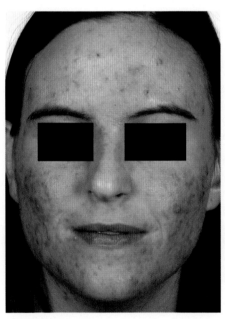

Figure 67.1

Questions

- What is the likely diagnosis?
- What is the underlying pathophysiology?
- What treatment would you suggest?

This patient had been suffering from acne vulgaris on her face for many years. This is a common condition, which usually starts around puberty but can persist into the third or fourth decades. Acne lesions develop from sebaceous glands that produce lipid material called sebum. Blockage of the sebaceous glands results in comedomes, which appear as small monomorphic papules, often on the forehead and cheeks. Comedomes can be closed (whiteheads) or open (blackheads) and are usually the primary acne lesions. In addition, there is increased sebum production and numbers of *Proprionibacterium acnes* bacteria within the ducts, which leads to inflammation around the glands. Painful cysts can then form which may heal with scarring.

Various factors are known to play a role in the development of acne including androgens, testosterone, oestrogens, sweating, occlusive oils and steroids. Women may develop acne as part of the polycystic ovarian syndrome. The impact of acne on a patient's well-being should not be underestimated. Many acne patients lose self-confidence and feel depressed as a consequence of their highly visible skin disease. Patients should therefore be treated early and effectively.

Most patients start on the acne treatment ladder with topical therapies (antibiotics, retinoids, benzoyl peroxide), and then progress to systemic treatment with antibiotics (tetracyclines, erythromycin), hormone preparations (females) and finally isotretinoin.

Isotretinoin is a vitamin A-derived medication, which is highly effective at treating and usually 'curing' acne through its action of shrinking-down the sebaceous glands by 90 per cent. Despite its high efficacy it is usually reserved for treating resistant or severe acne owing to its unfavourable side-effect profile.

Isotretinoin is teratogenic (90 per cent risk of birth defects). Therefore, women of childbearing age who are sexually active need a reliable form of contraception. The reduction in sebum production means patients taking the medication may suffer from severely dry lips and skin. Other side effects include a temporary rise in liver enzymes and lipids. Mood change and depression are potential side effects and therefore care should be taken when prescribing the medication to those with a history of depression or mental illness.

Patients usually take a cumulative target dose of isotretinoin between 120 and 150 mg/kg body weight over six to nine months. Most patients benefit from long-term elimination of their acne.

Residual scarring may be treated with topical retinoids, chemical peels, laser resurfacing and tiny pinch-grafts.

 KEY POINTS

- Acne is a common condition affecting up to 80 per cent of Western populations.
- Acne lesions include comedomes, papules, pustules, cysts and eventually scarring.
- Isotretinoin is a highly effective treatment for acne but needs careful prescribing and monitoring.

History

A 59-year-old man attends the dermatology clinic for a skin review following renal transplantation for hypertensive nephropathy. He is immunosuppressed with sirolimus and mycophenolate mofetil. He has a few viral warts on his hands but his main complaint is a 6-month history of facial redness and painful 'spots'. The erythema is exacerbated by heat. He has applied a bland emollient cream and topical antibacterials to the affected areas with little benefit. At the initial consultation he is noted to have a florid facial erythema with multiple papules and pustules over his forehead and cheeks. He is commenced on oral minocycline 100 mg daily and is asked to come back in 3 months.

Examination

On review after 3 months of minocycline his facial eruption is starting to improve but he has persistent erythema, papules and pustules; he is also noted to have a slate grey colour starting to appear on his nose (Fig. 68.1).

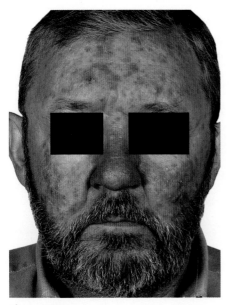

Figure 68.1

Questions

- What is the initial cutaneous diagnosis?
- What is the cause of the grey pigmentation on his nose?
- How would you now manage this patient?

This renal transplantation patient was suffering from florid rosacea that was unresponsive to topical therapy. He was treated with oral minocycline with some improvement in his rosacea after a few months. Rosacea is an acneiform condition that causes facial flushing, fixed erythema, papules, pustules and cutaneous oedema. If the tissue swelling becomes chronic then rhinophyma can result. Patients usually report an exacerbation of their condition with heat, spicy food and alcohol. Their erythematous skin tends to be sensitive and numerous topical preparations can cause burning or stinging.

Oral tetracyclines are usually highly effective in the treatment of rosacea. However, this patient developed slate-grey pigmentation on his nose secondary to the minocycline antibiotic. Of patients taking minocycline 3.7 per cent are reported to develop some altered skin pigmentation, usually within five months of commencing the treatment. The development of minocycline-induced pigmentation is not dose dependent. In many but not in all cases the slate-grey pigmentation fades eventually on discontinuation of the minocycline. This patient's minocycline was stopped and he was switched to oral lymecycline 408 mg daily which was effective in treating his rosacea.

The patient was given some sun-protection advice as tetracyclines can be photosensitizing. In addition patients who are post-transplantation and on immunosuppressive drugs are at an increased risk of skin cancer, therefore skin surveillance and sun-protection are paramount.

 KEY POINTS

- Rosacea is an acne-like condition with pustules and papules but also erythema and flushing.
- A side effect of oral minocycline is a slate-grey pigmentation in the skin, which may be permanent.
- Post-transplant patients on immunosuppressive medication are at increased risk of skin cancer.

History

A 5-year-old boy presents to the accident and emergency department with a sudden-onset facial eruption over the previous 24 hours. Initially the skin was erythematous and crusted, then his parents noticed blisters developing and were understandably concerned. Apart from a fever the previous day he is otherwise well, and is eating and drinking normally. He is recovering from a recent episode of chickenpox but otherwise has had no previous skin problems. No one else at home is obviously affected.

Examination

There are crusted resolving chickenpox lesions on his face, trunk and limbs. On his central face there are acute tense bullae and areas of golden crusting (Fig. 69.1), but no ulcers or erosions. Calamine lotion applied to the skin by his parents has given him a patchy white appearance. Elsewhere on the trunk and limbs there are healing crusted lesions and post-inflammatory hyperpigmentation. He is now apyrexial and has normal blood pressure and pulse rate.

 INVESTIGATIONS

Full blood count, renal and liver function tests were normal.
Skin swabs were taken for microbiology and virology cultures.

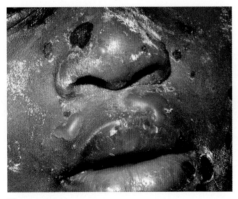

Figure 69.1

Questions

- Why do blisters form?
- What is the differential diagnosis?
- Who else may be affected?

Blisters (vesicles and bullae) are usually a sign of an acute cutaneous reaction. Blisters comprise clear, serous fluid, which may become cloudy due to the accumulation of neutrophils (pus), or blood-stained due to vascular damage. Blisters can form due to damage to the adhesion structures in between cells; this damage can result from friction/pressure, heat, infections, autoimmune-mediated complexes, phototoxic reactions, adverse drug reactions, and congenital deficiencies or malfunction of adhesion structures within the skin. Blisters can also form due to cutaneous oedema.

This child has bullous impetigo, which results from a cutaneous infection with exotoxin-producing strains of *Staphylococcus aureus* (confirmed by skin swabs). Exotoxins cause loss of cell–cell adhesion in the epidermis, resulting in superficial blisters which break down, leaving denuded areas and classic golden crusting. Impetigo is very common, especially in children, and is highly contagious with spread by direct inoculation. The initial infection may occur through a small break in the skin – this child had resolving chickenpox lesions which left his skin vulnerable to secondary bacterial infection. Other family members are commonly subsequently infected by contact with the index case.

Classically, impetigo develops rapidly on localized areas of skin. Blisters, pustules, erosions and golden crusted exudate complete the clinical picture. Patients are usually otherwise well. Skin swabs may isolate *S. aureus* or occasionally Streptococcus (group A).

Localized cutaneous impetigo can be managed with topical antiseptics such as dilute chlorhexidine to wash the skin and topical antibiotics such as fusidic acid, polymyxin or mupirocin. Oral antibiotics such as flucloxacillin or erythromycin may be required if involvement is more widespread.

 KEY POINTS

- Blisters indicate an acute cutaneous reaction.
- Impetigo is common and highly contagious.
- Patients with localized disease may be managed with topical antibiotics.

History

A 50-year-old woman presents to the accident and emergency department with a 2-day history of painful facial swelling that was unresponsive to chlorpheniramine. She had seen her GP 1-day previously who prescribed flucloxacillin 500 mg qds; however, over the next day the pain and swelling had worsened. On direct questioning she thinks she may have been stung by an insect 3 days ago on her left cheek. The eruption is not pruritic. She has no known allergies.

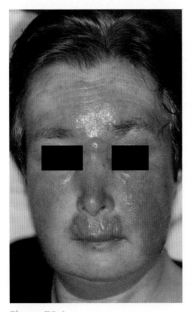

Examination

There is a well-demarcated, confluent, livid erythema with oedema and bullae formation, mainly on the left side of her face but spreading to the right (Fig. 70.1). There is no evidence of any skin erosions, no mucous membrane involvement and her vision is unaffected. She is apyrexial. Her blood pressure is 134/89 mmHg, pulse rate 92 /min, oxygen saturation on air 97%, blood sugar level on finger prick testing 7.9 mmol/L.

Figure 70.1

INVESTIGATIONS

		Normal
White cell count	17.04×10^9/L	$4.00–11.0 \times 10^9$/L
Haemoglobin	13.9 g/dL	11.5–16.5 g/dL
Platelets	326×10^9/L	$150–450 \times 10^9$/L
Neutrophils	14.81×10^9/L	$2.20–6.30 \times 10^9$/L
Lymphocytes	1.35×10^9/L	$1.30–4.00 \times 10^9$/L
Eosinophils	0.0×10^9/L	$0–0.4 \times 10^9$/L
C-reactive protein	292 mg/L	< 5 mg/L
Erythrocyte sedimentation rate	50 mm/h	1–13 mm/h

Renal and liver function tests were normal. Blood cultures were negative.

The skin swab was found to be negative for bacteriological and viral cultures.

Questions

- What is the diagnosis?
- What is the likely underlying cause?
- What treatment would you initiate?

This patient was diagnosed clinically with erysipelas. This is a cutaneous infection, usually caused on the face by group A *Streptococcus pyogenes*, which may originate from the patient's throat. The history of a possible insect bite was not thought to be significant but any minor skin laceration would act as a port of entry to microorganisms. The spread of the erythema is characteristically rapid and well demarcated (you could outline the edge with a skin marker); this contrasts with cellulitis, which usually has a slower onset with ill-defined margins. Cellulitis is deep, erysipelas is more superficial. Erysipelas may also affect the lower limb. The confluent erythema is very oedematous and consequently vesicles or bullae may form.

The differential diagnosis of sudden-onset facial erythema includes 'slapped cheek' or fifth disease, however this usually occurs in children, is symmetrical, and there is little oedema and no blistering. An acute allergic reaction usually presents more rapidly over a few hours rather than days and usually results from ingesting an allergen; such patients usually have lip swelling and may have gastrointestinal upset.

Patients with erysipelas should be managed initially with intravenous antibiotics. This patient was given 1.2 g benzylpenicillin and 2 g flucloxacillin qds for 2 days. The large bullae were deflated using a sterile needle. Gauze soaked in diluted potassium permanganate solution was applied to the affected skin once daily and topical fusidic acid applied. The patient was discharged on oral amoxicillin 1 g tds for 2 weeks.

 KEY POINTS

- Erysipelas characteristically affects the face or lower limb.
- The onset or erysipelas is rapid over 48 hours with well-demarcated erythema.
- Group A Streptococcus is usually the cause and should be treated initially with intravenous antibiotics.

History

A 55-year-old woman presents to the accident and emergency department with a 6-day history of swelling of her right lower leg. She has been finding it increasingly difficult to walk due to the pain. She does not recall any preceding trauma to her leg, and she has not recently travelled. She has no respiratory symptoms and has not had a temperature. There is no history of previous skin problems. She is otherwise fit and well.

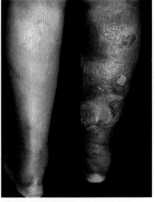

Figure 71.1

Examination

The right leg is hot, swollen and erythematous with indistinct borders (Fig. 71.1). Blisters are forming at the margins of the involved skin and several have broken down leaving eroded areas, which are weeping. There is no evidence of yellow crusting. The leg is tender to touch and there is pitting oedema to the knee. She has tender lymphadenopathy in the right inguinal region.

🔍 INVESTIGATIONS

		Normal
White cell count	11.31×10^9/L	4.00–11.0×10^9/L
Haemoglobin	12.6 g/dL	11.5–16.5 g/dL
Platelets	278×10^9/L	150–450×10^9/L
Neutrophils	8.34×10^9/L	2.20–6.30×10^9/L
Lymphocytes	2.30×10^9/L	1.30–4.00×10^9/L
C-reactive protein	254 mg/L	< 5 mg/L
Glucose	5.6 mmol/L	3.0–11.0 mmol/L
Sodium	135 mmol/L	135–145 mmol/L
Potassium	3.5 mmol/L	3.5–5.0 mmol/L
Creatinine	90 μmol/L	45–120 μmol/L
Urea	4.8 mmol/L	3.3–6.7 mmol/L
Albumin	44 g/L	35–50 g/L
Alkaline phosphatase	150 IU/L	30–130 IU/L
Aspartate transaminase	58 IU/L	10–50 IU/L
γ-glutamyl transferase	99 IU/L	1–55 IU/L
INR (international normalized ratio)	1.04	0.90–1.20
Duplex scan of the right leg	No thrombus seen above the knee, poor views in the calf due to excessive oedema, cannot rule out deep vein thrombosis	
Swab (right leg) microbiology	No significant growth	

Questions

- What is the most likely diagnosis?
- What organism might you expect to be the cause?
- What management would you implement?

This patient has cellulitis of the right leg. She has the classic signs of erythema, heat, swelling and local tenderness. Oedema blisters developed on the involved skin secondary to acute tissue swelling. The fragile blisters rapidly de-roofed (loss of the overlying epidermis) leaving eroded areas. Her duplex scan of the right lower leg was technically challenging due to the marked oedema, so thrombus could not be ruled out. However, the clinical signs were most in keeping with infection rather than thrombus. Occasionally patients have tender regional lymphadenopathy and a fever.

A swab taken from the involved skin was negative for microorganisms, which is typical in cellulitis as the infection is in the dermis and subcutis. Blood cultures are usually negative as most patients do not develop a bacteraemia. The cutaneous infection triggers an inflammatory response, which leads to the clinical signs of localized erythema, swelling, heat and tenderness.

As with most cases of lower leg cellulitis there was no history of trauma or preceding skin disease in this case. Occasionally patients may have tinea pedis (fungal infection) between their toes, which can act as a portal of entry to bacteria.

Cellulitis is most commonly caused by group A Streptococci or *Staphylococcus aureus*. *Streptococcus pneumoniae* can cause a very severe cellulitis of the leg, presenting with haemorrhagic bullae and necrosis, usually in immunocompromised patients or those with diabetes. *S. pneumoniae* may also cause cellulitis of the face as can *Haemophilus influenzae* type B.

Patients with moderate or severe cellulitis should be treated with intravenous antibiotics, usually in hospital. Benzylpenicillin, cephalosporins or macrolides can be given. Initially patients should rest, elevate their legs and be given suitable analgesia. Topical treatment may include potassium permanganate soaks, deflation of tense blisters, applications of topical antibiotics (to prevent secondary bacterial colonization) to any eroded areas and gentle compression to reduce the oedema.

 KEY POINTS

- Cellulitis is usually unilateral, the leg is hot, swollen, erythematous and tender.
- Skin swabs and blood cultures are usually negative for microbiological culture.
- Intravenous antibiotics are usually required plus elevation of the leg and light compression.

History

A 4-year-old girl is admitted to hospital with painful raw areas in her axillae, neck and groin. These have developed over 24 hours. Her skin had initially become erythematous and inflamed before peeling off to leave large superficial eroded areas in her flexures. She has a history of atopic eczema but is otherwise well. Her mother had suffered recurrent boils on the lower legs following varicose vein surgery one year previously but her skin was currently clear. The patient has not travelled abroad and does not have contact with animals. She does have intermittent contact with a childminder and other young children.

Examination

On admission the child looks unwell and is in pain, and her temperature is 38.3 °C. She holds her arms away from her body. Skin inspection reveals erythema and desquamation in her axillae (Fig. 72.1), groin (Fig. 72.2) and around her neck. She has moderate eczema on her limb flexures. Her mucous membranes are normal.

🔍 INVESTIGATIONS

Swabs were taken from the groin and axillae.
Blood tests were normal.

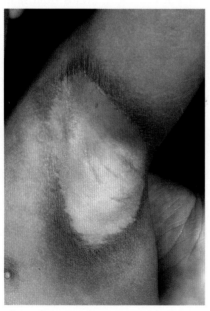

Figure 72.1

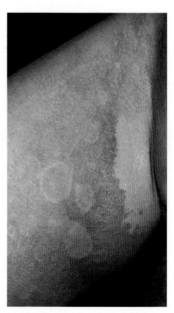

Figure 72.2

Questions

- What is the clinical diagnosis?
- What are the swabs likely to isolate?
- How would you treat this patient?

This child looked unwell and had tender skin. There was extensive erythema and desquamation in her groin and axillae leading to a diagnosis of staphylococcal scalded skin syndrome (SSSS). This is an exfoliative toxin-mediated bacterial infection mainly affecting children under the age of 5 years. Flexural areas of skin are classically involved; however, the cutaneous involvement may become widespread. Children may have suffered a recent bacterial infection of their ear or throat. Children with atopic eczema are frequently colonized by *Staphylococcus aureus*, of which 5 per cent of strains produce exotoxins which are spread through the blood leading to widespread skin involvement by SSSS.

Children may be pyrexial and appear unwell; they do not want their skin to be touched at the affected sites owing to tenderness/pain. Lateral pressure on affected skin can lead to a positive Nikolsky's sign (the superficial skin sloughs-off). Swabs from involved skin usually isolate *S. aureus*; strain typing and identification of exotoxins can be carried out if the diagnosis is in doubt. Interestingly, blood cultures are usually negative in children. This child's skin swabs also isolated *Pseudomonas*, which is an opportunistic secondary colonizer of eroded skin.

The patient was admitted to hospital and treated with oral flucloxacillin (intravenous lines should be avoided in patients with fragile/infected skin if possible) plus topical combination fusidic acid and hydrocortisone. She washed in a mild chlorhexidine lotion as the pain settled.

This child had several episodes of SSSS over a few months. Swabs from family members and close contacts were negative for *S. aureus* nasal carriage. The patient therefore required a prolonged course of oral flucloxacillin to try to prevent relapse. She was also treated with clindamycin, which inhibits exotoxin formation by *S. aureus*. The *Pseudomonas* was treated with ciprofloxacin as it was felt in this case that the bacterium was having a significant secondary impact on slow skin healing. Mild topical hydrogen peroxide cream was also used as a local antiseptic.

 KEY POINTS

- Staphylococcal scalded skin syndrome (SSSS) usually occurs in children under the age of 5 years.
- Erythema and desquamation, especially in the flexures, is common with SSSS and may be widespread.
- Systemic and topical antibiotics plus antiseptic washes usually settle the condition over a few weeks.

History

A 32-year-old actor presents to the accident and emergency department with a 7-day history of malaise, fever, aching in his joints and neck, and a persistent headache. He has also noticed a rash on his palms and soles and is worried that he might have developed meningitis. He had eczema as a child but otherwise no previous skin problems. He takes antihistamines for hay fever. He lives alone and has no significant past medical history. The casualty officer arranges for some preliminary blood tests and asks for a dermatological opinion on the skin eruption.

Examination

There are multiple, small erythematous macules 1–4 mm in diameter and patches with mild superficial scale on his palms (Fig. 73.1) and plantar aspect of his feet (Fig. 73.2). Some of the lesions are slightly pigmented and there is some desquamation in places. He has a few similar lesions scattered over his trunk. The lesions are blanching. His mucous membranes, scalp and nails are normal. He has mild neck stiffness but no photophobia and his temperature is 38.0 °C.

 INVESTIGATIONS

Blood tests results were requested.

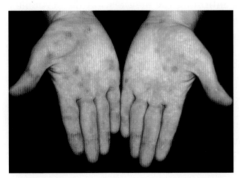

Figure 73.1

Questions

- What is the clinical diagnosis?
- What tests would you need to perform to confirm the diagnosis?
- How would you manage this patient?

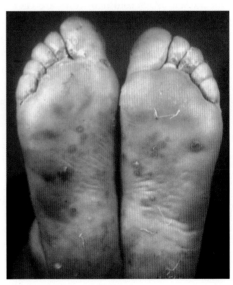

Figure 73.2

Fever, headache and a rash is a common combination of symptoms with a wide differential diagnosis. Many viral infections such as measles, chickenpox, Epstein–Barr virus and viral meningitis can present in this way. This patient was concerned about bacterial meningitis but the rash was blanching and not purpuric. The diagnosis is secondary syphilis, which can be easily missed. The rash of secondary syphilis is frequently subtle and asymptomatic in most cases. Patients develop non-specific symptoms of malaise and may not present to a medical practitioner.

The rash of secondary syphilis classically affects the palms, soles and trunk, but may become widespread. Lesions start as small erythematous papules and macules that may become slightly scaly and form erythematous-to-pigmented patches. The eruption is usually asymptomatic and may be misdiagnosed as guttate psoriasis. Patients usually develop 'flu-like' or even 'meningitis-like' symptoms. The rash of secondary syphilis usually appears 1–3 months following the initial infection. The spirochete *Treponema pallidum* is usually transmitted by sexual intercourse and at the site of entry a small painless ulcer (chancre) appears on the genitals/mouth.

If syphilis remains untreated a tertiary stage affecting several organ systems can develop many years later. Classically, the central nervous system is affected leading to mental disturbance and even dementia, spinal cord involvement leads to sensory neuropathy and autonomic dysfunction of the bladder. Cutaneous manifestations at this late stage include nodules (gummas) which may ulcerate.

Early diagnosis is essential to ensure long-term sequelae are avoided and the infection is not passed on. Serological tests are the key to confirming the diagnosis at the secondary syphilis stage. Specific treponemal antibody tests include TPHA (*T. pallidum* haemagglutination) and TPPA (*T. pallidum* particle agglutination), which can confirm infection with syphilis. However, the exact timing of disease acquisition may only be estimated owing to rising or falling titres of non-specific tests such as VDRL (Venereal Disease Research Laboratory) and RPR (rapid plasma regain). The latter usually becomes negative after effective treatment whereas TPHA remains positive for life.

If patients present with a chancre, then a smear can be taken onto a glass slide for darkfield immunofluorescence microscopy to identify the spirochaetes. Patients should also undergo a full sexual health screen and be offered an HIV test, as the two diseases may be transmitted simultaneously.

Treatment of early disease is with intramuscular benzathine penicillin G 2.4 million units in a single dose, and for late disease is four times weekly for 3 weeks. Use of ceftriaxone and azithromycin is currently being evaluated but appears highly effective. For penicillin-sensitive patients doxycycline has been traditionally prescribed 100 mg daily for 14 days (increased to 30 days in late disease and 200 mg daily for 30 days for neurosyphilis).

 KEY POINTS

- The incidence of syphilis worldwide is increasing and may be simultaneously transmitted with HIV.
- The rash of secondary syphilis may be subtle with palmar/plantar red/brown scaly macules/patches.
- A combination of serological tests is usually needed to confirm the disease and the stage.

History

A 10-year-old boy presents to the accident and emergency department with a 7-day history of a blister, which appeared on his lower lip with subsequent crusting and is now spreading over the right side of his cheek. He complains of pain in his mouth, lip and right side of his face, which feels swollen. He is initially referred to the maxillary-facial team with a suspected dental abscess. An orthopantomogram X-ray is normal; he is then referred to the on-call dermatology team. He reports an allergy to erythromycin.

Examination

He has tense blistering and erythematous crusted lesions on his right lower lip and cheek (Fig. 74.1). There is erythema that has golden crusting with vesiculation particularly on his lower lip. He has tender lymphadenopathy in the supraclavicular region. Inside his mouth there is no evidence of a dental abscess.

🔎 INVESTIGATIONS

Swabs were taken for microbiological and virological analysis.

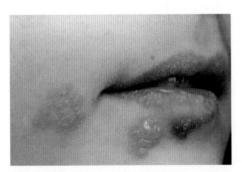

Figure 74.1

Questions

- What is the most likely diagnosis?
- What secondary cutaneous complication has arisen?
- How would you manage this patient acutely and in the future?

When any patient presents with a blistering eruption on the lip, the most likely diagnosis is herpes simplex virus (HSV), usually type I. Patients may describe a prodrome of tingling and pain 24–48 hours prior to the onset of blistering. Although the lip is the most common site (herpes labialis), lesions of HSV can occur at other mucous membrane sites (nose and genitalia, usually type II), or indeed anywhere else on the skin.

Primary HSV is usually asymptomatic, however in a small minority of patients the initial infection can be very severe and extensive. Subsequent attacks occur due to reactivation of the life-long persistent HSV, which stays within the dorsal root ganglion of the affected nerve. Attacks of so-called 'cold-sores' can occur at intervals, usually at the same mucous membrane/skin site. Triggers include cold weather, bright sunlight, immunosuppression, intercurrent illness, trauma and high altitude.

The differential diagnosis of blistering on the lips includes primary impetigo, burn/ trauma, hand-foot and mouth, erythema multiforme major, Stevens–Johnson syndrome, toxic epidermal necrolysis, fixed drug eruption, immunobullous disease and porphyria. The history, clinical signs and investigations should, however, help to distinguish HSV from these other diagnoses.

This patient suffered a HSV type I infection of the right lower lip and subsequently developed secondary impetigo due to *Staphylococcus aureus* (an 'aureus' was a gold coin issued in Rome in the first century BC). Secondary bacterial infection is particularly common with HSV infections and is characterized by golden crusted areas on the skin. Antibacterial washes containing low concentrations of chlorhexidine (Dermol®) are helpful in clearing mild, localized skin infections. Topical (fucidin) or oral antibiotics (flucloxacillin, erythromycin) are required in some cases.

Swabs that were sent to the laboratory in viral transport medium confirmed the presence of HSV type I DNA. If patients present within 72 hours of the onset of HSV infections, then a course of oral aciclovir is helpful. Patients can purchase topical aciclovir over the counter, which can be effective in mild attacks if treated early. Patients developing recurrent symptomatic attacks may benefit from secondary prophylaxis with aciclovir 400 mg daily, other patients may prefer to have some aciclovir tablets at home to take immediately they become symptomatic with the prodrome/blisters.

 KEY POINTS

- Herpes simplex virus (HSV) reactivation is usually preceded by a cutaneous prodrome of tingling and pain.
- Recurrent attacks of blistering affecting a mucous membrane site are likely to be caused by HSV.
- Patients suffering from recurrent attacks of reactivation may require secondary prophylaxis with aciclovir.

History

A 69-year-old retired man is referred by his GP to the on-call dermatology registrar with a 1-week history of increasing pain, erythema and blisters on the left side of his face. He is unable to open his left eye. Two days prior to the onset of the cutaneous eruption the patient had complained of pain on swallowing and pain in the left ear and temple area, when he was prescribed flucloxacillin. He has a history of hypertension and is taking amlodipine and simvastatin.

Examination

He has marked swelling of the left side of his face with prominent periorbital oedema (Fig. 75.1). There is a sticky discharge around his left eye. He has multiple vesicles on a background of erythema with crusting and erosions. There is a small area of ulceration on the lower lip with multiple ulcers on the hard palate and buccal mucosa. The signs and symptoms are localized to the left side of his face. His temperature is 37.8 °C, blood pressure 133/78 mmHg and pulse rate 67 beats/min.

INVESTIGATIONS

		Normal
C-reactive protein	30.2 mg/L	< 5.0 mg/L
Erythrocyte sedimentation rate	23 mm/h	< 10 mm/h

The urine dipstick tests were negative.
A viral swab was taken.

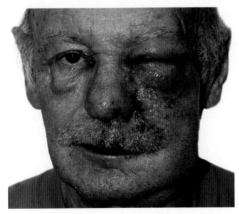

Figure 75.1

Questions
- What is the diagnosis?
- What is the source of his infection?
- How would you manage this patient?

This man had herpes zoster virus (HZV) (shingles) affecting the left mandibular branch of the trigeminal nerve. The first symptom is usually tingling followed by severe pain in the skin supplied by the affected nerve. Patients feel unwell and may develop localized tender lymphadenopathy. Within a few days a localized cutaneous eruption occurs in crops of erythematous papules that rapidly form into blisters which then crust over and heal with scarring over a few weeks.

The patient will have acquired HZV from a primary chickenpox infection (usually in childhood) after which the virus remains latent in the spinal dorsal root ganglia. When the virus is reactivated (most frequently in the elderly) as shingles the cutaneous dermatome supplied by the sensory nerve is affected. In this case the mandibular branch of the trigeminal nerve was affected resulting in cutaneous/mucocutaneous signs in the distribution of the nerve (supplying the skin of the temporal region, lower lip and chin, buccal mucosa, muscles of mastication, mucous membrane of the anterior two-thirds of the tongue). Sensory nerve involvement is characteristic of shingles; however, 5 per cent of cases include motor nerve involvement. Multi-dermatomal shingles is seen in immunocompromised patients.

If possible, patients should receive aciclovir within 72 hours of the onset of the cutaneous eruption. Oral aciclovir is sufficient for the majority of patients (800 mg five times daily for 7–10 days). However, this patient developed severe oral ulceration and pain on swallowing and therefore was treated with intravenous aciclovir (5 mg/kg body weight, three times a day) for the first 48 hours of his treatment followed by a further 7 days of oral therapy. Consider intravenous therapy if there is involvement of the eye, motor nerves or if the patient is immunocompromised. If motor involvement is severe, consider giving oral prednisolone in addition to aciclovir.

The cutaneous eruption should be treated topically with an emollient such as 50:50 white soft paraffin with liquid paraffin (hourly if necessary) to keep the affected skin greasy. The emollient helps reduce pain in the eroded areas and the likelihood of fissures (skin splitting) as the blisters crust over. The emollient also acts as a barrier to help prevent secondary bacterial infection in the denuded areas of skin. Topical antibiotic ointments may be indicated if secondary infection is suspected. Occasionally oral antibiotics may be indicated.

This patient was jointly managed with the ophthalmologists who recommended regular eyelid cleaning with sterile normal saline and chloramphenicol 1% ointment four times daily to the left eye. Analgesia (such as non-steroidal anti-inflammatory drugs) should be given in the acute phase and for post-herpetic neuralgia, which may be severe and protracted (consider gabapentin or amitriptyline).

 KEY POINTS

- Treatment with antiviral drugs should be started as early as possible to improve clinical outcomes.
- Topical treatment to the skin and affected mucous membranes helps reduce pain and complications.
- Multi-dermatomal zoster should alert the clinician to a patient with underlying immunosuppression.

History

A 38-year-old woman is admitted to hospital with a 6-week history of increasing shortness of breath on exertion, fever, dry cough, malaise and weight loss. She also complains of multiple 'spots' on her face and chest, which have become more numerous over the past 2 weeks. Her past medical history is unremarkable and she has no history of previous skin problems. She has been taking paracetamol for her fevers, but otherwise is not on any regular medication.

Examination

She looks unwell and is breathless at rest, her temperature is 38.5 °C; chest examination reveals mild crackles in the mid zones only. On her skin she has multiple, small (2-3 mm in diameter), firm, flesh-coloured papules on her face (Fig. 76.1) and chest. Many of the papules have a central umbilicated depression, the surrounding skin is normal.

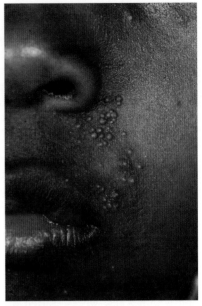

Figure 76.1

🔍 INVESTIGATIONS

Chest X-ray showed bilateral diffuse patchy infiltrates in the mid zones. Bronchoalveolar lavage samples were sent for microscopy and culture.

Questions

- What is the skin diagnosis?
- What is the respiratory diagnosis?
- What is the unifying underlying diagnosis?

When patients present with a cutaneous eruption in association with other signs or symptoms, the skin can often give a vital clue to the underlying/unifying diagnosis. Skin can be the 'window' to internal disease. This patient had very characteristic skin lesions of molluscum contagiosum. The flesh-coloured umbilicated papules are caused by a cutaneous infection with a highly contagious poxvirus. Gently squeezing an individual lesion characteristically causes the extrusion of semi-solid white material (comprising the molluscum bodies). Poxvirus is spread by direct contact and autoinoculation is common. When adults present with multiple lesions, then underlying immune compromise should be suspected. Molluscum contagiosum in young children is seen in otherwise healthy individuals.

This patient was found to be HIV-positive with a viral load of 632 000 copies/mL and a CD4 lymphocyte count of 3. It is estimated that approximately 10 per cent of adult HIV patients have molluscum contagiosum and that the more widespread the lesions, the lower their CD4 lymphocyte count.

The patient's progressive respiratory symptoms were caused by co-infection with *Pneumocystis* (*carinii*) *jiroveci* and *Mycobacterium tuberculosis* pneumonia. This dual respiratory infection is not uncommon in patients from sub-Saharan Africa.

The patient immediately received treatment for her acute pneumonia and tuberculosis and within a few weeks started on HAART (highly active antiretroviral therapy). After discharge from hospital she was seen in the dermatology out-patient clinic and had the molluscum lesions treated fortnightly with cryotherapy (liquid nitrogen). The molluscum slowly cleared with a combination of cryotherapy and immune reconstitution.

Molluscum contagiosum is usually self-resolving in children and those with an intact immune system. Inflammation around the lesions is usually seen just prior to their resolution indicating activation of the patient's own immune system in dealing with the cutaneous infection. Most attempts at treating molluscum lesions revolve around destructive/ irritant methods, such as with acid chemicals, cryotherapy and immunotherapy (topical imiquimod 5% cream daily).

 KEY POINTS

- Multiple molluscum contagiosum lesions in an adult may indicate underlying immunodeficiency.
- Molluscum contagiosum is a poxvirus spread by direct contact and is not uncommon in children.
- Molluscum is self-resolving, but locally destructive treatments may speed resolution.

History

A 51-year-old patient under the care of the haematologists is referred to the dermatology clinic with a 6-year history of multiple papules and nodules on her fingers. The lesions have slowly been increasing in size and number over the last two years and are mainly asymptomatic. The lesions were treated with liquid nitrogen by her GP but they were unresponsive. She had been diagnosed two years previously with stage B chronic lymphocytic leukaemia (CLL). She has received several courses of chlorambucil, fludarabine and cyclophosphamide to which she partially responded and is being considered for alemtuzumab (Campath – antiCD52) biological therapy in the future.

Examination

She has multiple hyperkeratotic flesh-coloured papules and nodules, mainly over the dorsi of her fingers and hands (Fig. 77.1) The lesions are warty in nature and firm on palpation. The surrounding skin is normal.

INVESTIGATIONS

At the time of review in the dermatology clinic, blood counts were normal.

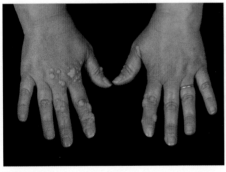

Figure 77.1

Questions

- Why does she have multiple lesions on her hands?
- What treatment options are possible for her skin lesions?

This woman has been suffering from multiple viral warts on her hands for many years. The warts result from an infection with human papilloma virus (HPV) in the cutaneous keratinocytes. HPV is specific to humans and is passed by direct skin contact and through fomites. HPV infects the basal keratinocytes; when these infected cells leave the basal layer they become highly differentiated, triggering viral genome replication. Consequently, when the keratinocytes reach the epithelial surface, viral particles are released with the sloughed-off cells into the environment where they can survive for many months.

HPV infections are common in the general population but are more frequently found in patients who are immunosuppressed, when warts are often multiple. CLL causes down-regulation of immune surveillance and an increased susceptibility to all manner of infections. In addition, chemotherapy depletes patients' white cell populations rendering them more vulnerable to infections. These patients are unable to clear the HPV and subsequently develop multiple recalcitrant warts.

Although cutaneous warts are not harmful in themselves they can cause a considerable amount of distress to patients both psychologically and socially. Patients frequently feel embarrassed by their warts and can often feel stigmatized by others.

Most treatments for HPV are locally destructive (cryotherapy with liquid nitrogen, salicylic acid, electrodessication, CO_2 laser) and then the host's immune cells 'mop-up' the residual virus released; however, when the host's immune system is suboptimal, locally destructive treatments are frequently ineffective.

Although not licensed to treat cutaneous warts, treatment options include immunotherapy with imiquimod 5% cream (daily with Elastoplast occlusion) or diphencyprone (DPC) fortnightly. DPC is a highly sensitizing chemical – patients are rendered allergic to it by painting a small amount on their forearm skin, then increasing percentages are applied directly to the warts to recruit immune cells into the local tissue. Cure rates of 60 per cent are reported in immunosuppressed patients after 6 months of treatment. This patient was treated with DPC immunotherapy to good effect. Topical bleomycin has also been used with some success to treat recalcitrant warts in this group of patients.

 KEY POINTS

- If a patient presents with multiple HPV warts, then consider immune deficiency.
- Warts will eventually resolve spontaneously in the majority of patients.
- Management of warts includes local destructive modalities and immunotherapy to the skin.

History

A 42-year-old woman presents to the accident and emergency department with a 1-week history of malaise and a widespread rash that started on her face and spread distally. In addition she complains of a temperature, vomiting, diarrhoea, productive cough and painful red eyes. She has just finished a course of amoxicillin for recurrent sinusitis. Her two young children have recently had a viral illness with a rash. She was previously well with no underlying medical problems. She is admitted to a side room and referred to the dermatology team.

Examination

The patient is pyrexial with a temperature of 39.4 °C. She has an extensive erythematous maculopapular eruption, which is particularly marked on her face, neck and trunk (Fig. 78.1). Some of the papules are coalescing into plaques with central bullae. Examination of her mouth reveals marked erythema with prominent white spots on her palate and buccal mucosae (Fig. 78.2). Her conjunctivae are erythematous and injected.

INVESTIGATIONS

Chest X-ray showed right lower lobe consolidation.
Viral serology and oral fluid tests, sputum culture and skin biopsy were performed.

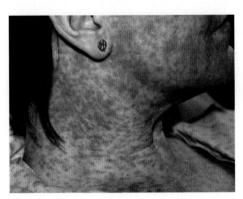

Figure 78.1

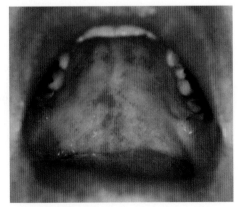

Figure 78.2

Questions

- What is the most likely diagnosis and possible complication?
- How would you confirm the diagnosis?
- Who else may need some form of treatment and what form should that take?

This woman was obviously unwell on admission. A viral illness was suspected but a possible reaction to amoxicillin was also considered. Oral fluid swab and serology confirmed a diagnosis of measles. Her two children had recently had a viral illness that was subsequently confirmed as measles. The patient herself had been partially vaccinated with MMR (measles, mumps, rubella) vaccine as a child. Measles is highly contagious and passes readily among contacts through droplet spread; the incubation period is 1–2 weeks.

Patients frequently experience a prodrome of fever and malaise with photophobia and conjunctivitis. White Koplik's spots on the buccal mucosa/palate are virtually pathognomonic, but not always present. The cutaneous eruption usually appears within days of the onset of symptoms, first appearing behind the ears and then spreading caudally. The rash is erythematous and mainly macular but can develop papules, which may coalesce and blister. Complications include otitis media, encephalitis and bronchopneumonia. This patient developed a chest infection as a complication of her measles; sputum culture grew *Haemophilus influenzae*.

Oral fluid can be collected using a foam swab and sent to the virology laboratory for rapid diagnosis of measles via RNA detection tests. IgM antibodies to measles can be detected around day 4 after the onset of the rash (90–100 per cent sensitivity) and up to 3 months thereafter. Mid-stream urine, nasopharyngeal and conjunctival swabs can also be taken to confirm the presence of measles virus.

Management of measles is largely supportive and patients should be isolated, so they don't transmit this highly infectious disease; however, patients may need admitting to hospital for treatment of any serious complications that may arise. Close contacts of those infected with measles are likely to develop the disease if they are not immune (through vaccination or previous infection). Measles is a notifiable disease in the United Kingdom so the local Consultant for Communicable Diseases should be informed.

Young children who have not yet been vaccinated but who have been exposed to measles can be given two doses of live attenuated MMR vaccine to try to prevent disease onset. Vitamin A supplementation during the acute illness has been shown to reduce morbidity and mortality.

 KEY POINTS

- Measles is highly contagious; patients are infectious 2 days prior to the onset of the rash.
- The maculopapular and erythematous rash spreads in a cephalocaudal direction.
- Patients with severe complications of measles may need treatment in hospital.

History

A 3-year-old boy is noted by his parents to have two small erythematous papules on his abdomen just before bedtime. The next morning he feels hot and has developed multiple lesions over his trunk, some of which look like blisters. Later that day he develops vomiting and diarrhoea and his parents take him to the accident and emergency department. The child has previously been well and attends nursery four days per week. No other family members are obviously affected. His mother feels tired as she is currently 12 weeks pregnant with her third child.

Examination

The child feels hot and looks slightly miserable, he does not obviously look dehydrated. There are multiple erythematous papules and vesicles over the child's abdomen (Fig. 79.1), back and around his neck. Most of the vesicles are intact, however some have ruptured and are starting to crust. There are a few excoriation marks around his neck. Mucous membranes are normal.

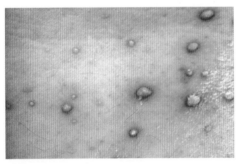

Figure 79.1

Questions

- What would be your first course of action?
- What is the most likely diagnosis?
- What investigations might be required?
- What treatment should be offered and to whom?

Chickenpox caused by varicella zoster virus (VZV) is a common, highly contagious infectious disease that usually affects young children. In the United States children are vaccinated against VZV to try to prevent the disease, however this is not routinely given in the United Kingdom as the disease is considered mild. It is also thought that the lower rates of shingles (latent reactivation of VZV in the skin) in adults who themselves had chickenpox as a child results from chronic exposure to the virus through contact with infected individuals. The virus is spread by droplets from the respiratory tract and from infected blister fluid (of chickenpox and shingles). There is usually a history of contact with another person with chickenpox/shingles 21 days before symptoms and signs develop. Patients are contagious 2 days prior to the onset of the rash and until all the lesions have completed crusted over.

Chickenpox can cause mild choryzal symptoms, headache, fever and even diarrhoea and vomiting. Small erythematous papules appear in clusters usually on the abdomen initially and then form blisters that appear in crops over a few days spreading outwards across the trunk and limbs. The lesions are classically at different stages: some papules, some blisters, and some crusted lesions starting to heal over. The eruption is usually itchy and many children scratch the tops off the vesicles, which can lead to scars that may be atrophic or keloid.

The first action you should take if assessing a child with potential chickenpox is to move out of the general waiting area/communal areas into a side room. VZV can be potentially serious if transmitted to non-immune, immunocompromised and pregnant individuals. It is important in this case to ascertain if the mother herself has previously had chickenpox as she is currently 12 weeks pregnant. Serology tests can look for rising titres of antibodies to VZV (IgM) in active disease and signs of life-long immunity (IgG) to VZV. Blister fluid can be analysed by polymerase chain reaction for the virus in those with the rash.

VZV acquisition in pregnancy can lead to maternal pneumonia, premature labour, and even maternal death. Fetuses and newborns infected with primary VZV often develop very severe disease. Non-immune pregnant women exposed to VZV should be given varicella zoster immune globulin within 96 hours of exposure.

Children with severe chickenpox – that is, 300–500 lesions on a background of atopic eczema – may occasionally need treatment with aciclovir. Mild topical steroids should be restarted once the lesions are starting to crust over to help reduce inflammation, exacerbation of eczema and possible scarring. VZV remains latent in the body for life in the sensory dorsal root ganglion where reactivation results in shingles in distribution of the sensory cutaneous nerve (dermatome). Acute shingles can be very painful and even after healing can result in post-herpetic neuralgia.

 KEY POINTS

- Chickenpox is caused by exposure to VSV and has an incubation period of 21 days.
- Crops of blisters appear on the trunk over several days.
- Non-immune at-risk individuals (pregnancy, immunocompromised) exposed to VZV may need aciclovir or zoster immune globulin.

History

A 54-year-old man with a 1-year history of multiple skin boils is seen in the dermatology clinic. These had started within two months of returning from India. The lesions first appeared as small red nodules, which increased in size and became painful before discharging pus. The lesions seemed to heal slowly, leaving scars. New lesions would then appear every few weeks. He has taken numerous courses of antibiotics from his GP, which seemed partially helpful, and has required incision and drainage of some of the larger, more painful furuncles. His wife, who is a nurse working in the local orthopaedics department, does not have any skin problems. The patient has a history of inflammatory bowel disease but is otherwise well and not taking any regular medications.

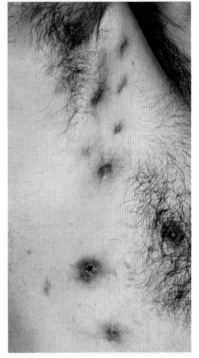

Figure 80.1

Examination

Multiple actively discharging boils and furuncles are seen on the right side of his chest with scarred areas from healed lesions (Fig. 80.1). He has a few boils elsewhere: on his left hip, and neck. There are palpable lymph nodes in the right axilla. Examination is otherwise unremarkable and his temperature is 37 °C.

🔍 INVESTIGATIONS

A swab was taken from the pus and carrier sites (nose, axilla, groin, throat) for microbiological analysis. Full blood count was normal.

Questions

- What organism is most likely the cause of his boils?
- Why might the boils not clear up with conventional systemic antibiotics?
- What special microbiological test would you request?

Recurrent recalcitrant boils caused by the bacterium *Staphylococcus aureus* are usually seen in young to middle-aged adults. Conventional treatment of large/painful furuncles is incision and drainage with 2 weeks of oral antibiotics. This patient, however, did not respond to this traditional approach. Pus from the active boils taken by the GP cultured methicillin-resistant *Staphylococcus aureus* (MRSA) – this was a hospital-acquired rather than the community-acquired type of MRSA.

Subsequently, swabs were taken in the dermatology department from the active lesions as well as his carrier sites and sent to the microbiology department with a special request for gene detection studies to look for *S. aureus* with the virulence factor Panton Valentine leukocidin (PVL). Microbiology results showed the patient to have MRSA and PVL-positive *S. aureus* in the boils and up his nose.

PVL is a virulence factor that is acquired by certain strains of *S. aureus* rendering them difficult to kill by conventional antibiotic treatment regimens. Not all strains that are PVL-positive are also resistant. In fact most are fully sensitive to methicillin; however bacteria that are resistant and virulent are very recalcitrant clinically and therapeutically, as in this case.

This patient may have acquired his PVL-positive *S. aureus* whilst travelling in India – travel is a risk factor for acquiring this virulent strain, as are contact sports and keeping pets. There was no direct evidence that the patient acquired the bacteria from his wife (who worked in hospitals) as her swabs were all negative. Nonetheless there is evidence that PVL-positive strains of *S. aureus* are also highly transmissible and this is thought to play a role in multiple family/team members being simultaneously affected.

Treatment for PVL-positive *S. aureus* is similar to treatment for MRSA, in that patients require decontamination therapy alongside systemic antibiotics. This patient was treated with nasal mupirocin three times a day for 5 days up each nostril. He was asked to wash daily with Hibiscrub (4% chlorhexidine). He was asked to take rifampicin and clindamycin 300 mg twice daily for 10 weeks. All the lesions healed and no new lesions appeared. Follow-up swabs from all sites were negative.

In patients with PVL-positive *S. aureus* that is fully sensitive to methicillin, a prolonged course of high-dose flucloxacillin plus decontamination may be sufficient to clear the infection. Asymptomatic family members should be swabbed, and if found to be positive at their carrier sites should also undergo decontamination.

 KEY POINTS

- Consider virulent strains of *Staphylococcus aureus* in patients with severe or recurrent boils.
- Ask your microbiologist to undertake special gene detection tests on *S. aureus* isolates to look for PVL.
- Patients should undertake decontamination with nasal antibiotic, antiseptic wash and prolonged courses of systemic antibiotics.

CASE 81: CHRONIC, SORE, MACERATED SKIN IN THE FINGER WEBS

History

A 46-year-old housewife with known multisystem sarcoidosis comes for a regular follow-up visit to the dermatology clinic. She complains of an increasing number of asymptomatic skin lesions on her limbs. She also mentions soreness between her fingers where the skin has started to break down. She had become increasingly breathless over the past two months and after consultation with the respiratory team she was commenced on a slowly reducing course of oral prednisolone and is currently taking 30 mg daily. Her past medical history includes hypothyroidism and idiopathic thrombocytopenic purpura.

Examination

She is slightly breathless at rest and looks mildly cushingoid. The skin between her fingers is erythematous with superficial white maceration (Fig. 81.1) and ulceration forming deep fissures (Fig. 81.2). In addition she has indurated, slightly hyperpigmented nodules and plaques on her limbs.

 INVESTIGATIONS

		Normal
Angiotensin converting enzyme	89 U/L	8–52 U/L

Chest X-ray shows bilateral hilar lymphadenopathy, with fibrotic changes in the lower and mid zones.

A finger web skin swab was taken.

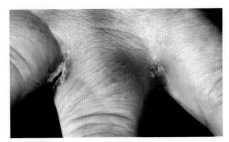

Figure 81.1

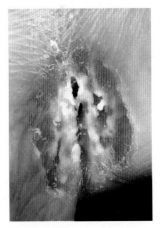

Figure 81.2

Questions

- What is the likely underlying cause of the skin changes in the finger webs?
- What is the cause of the cutaneous lesions on this patient's limbs?
- How would you manage her skin?

This patient has multiple, indurated, asymptomatic nodules and plaques of cutaneous sarcoidosis on her limbs. She had been taking systemic corticosteroids for her deteriorating respiratory sarcoid. This iatrogenic immunosuppression had left the patient vulnerable to infection. She developed a *Candida albicans* intertrigo in her finger webs (confirmed by yeast culture from her skin swab). This presentation is occasionally referred to as erosio interdigitalis blastomycetica (interdigital candidosis) and can be associated with occupations requiring frequent 'wet work' such as housework and gardening. Clinically, this superficial yeast infection is characterized by erythema, maceration and peeling of the flexural skin between the fingers. So-called 'satellite lesions' can often be seen as small erythematous papules/pustules at the periphery of the area of yeast-infected skin. *Candida* prefers a warm moist environment and hence the most commonly affected skin sites include the groin, natal cleft, axillae, under the breasts and between the digits.

C. albicans yeast forms part of normal human flora, with reservoirs in the gastrointestinal tract and vagina. *C. albicans* is not part of the normal skin flora, however it can transiently colonize flexural areas. The fine balance between the patient's immune system and yeast numbers can be easily upset by minor changes in the local skin environment, use of antibiotics, raised serum glucose and immune compromise through disease or medications leading to active candidiasis of the skin.

Management of *Candida* intertrigo includes trying to ensure the skin is kept as dry as possible to make the local skin environmentally hostile to the yeast. This can be achieved by using drying soaks such as potassium permanganate, antifungal powders and acetic acid. Antifungal treatments can be given orally or applied topically. Many dermatologists will try to manage localized disease with a topical combination antifungal cream plus anti-inflammatory steroid. Short courses of oral fluconazole or itraconazole may, however, be required in patients who are immunosuppressed or who have recalcitrant disease.

This patient needed to remain on her systemic corticosteroids and therefore oral fluconazole was given to try to help eliminate the *Candida* intertrigo over a few weeks. In addition she was asked to wash her hands once daily in chlorhexidine and to apply Canestan cream twice daily. This type of infection can take several weeks to clear, particularly in patients who are diabetic or immunosuppressed.

 KEY POINTS

- Cutaneous *Candida* infections should be suspected in flexural skin with erythema and maceration.
- *Candida* yeasts more frequently cause skin disease in patients who are vulnerable such as neonates, the immunocompromised and the elderly.
- Combination treatment with skin drying agents, antifungals and topical steroids are effective.

History

A 56-year-old Albanian man presents to the dermatology clinic with a 2-year history of developing asymptomatic purple lesions on his skin. The initial lesions appeared on his feet 4 months after an orthoptic liver transplant for hepatitis B. Over the past few months he has developed further cutaneous lesions on his legs, arms and trunk. He is taking systemic prednisolone and tacrolimus.

Examination

There are well-demarcated macular purple patches on his shoulder, forearms, dorsi of his hands, right calf and left foot. The lesions on the left foot and medial shin are indurated, firm plaques (Fig. 82.1). The mouth, genitals, scalp and nails are normal.

INVESTIGATIONS

A skin biopsy was taken from a lesion on the left foot.
An HIV test was carried out.
A computed tomography (CT) scan of the chest was performed.

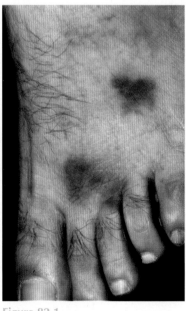

Figure 82.1

Questions

- What is the cause of the skin lesions?
- What is the aetiological agent?
- How would you manage this patient?

Cutaneous lesions with a vascular origin frequently appear as purple discolouration, including purpura, vasculitis, livedo, vascular occlusion (thrombosis) and vascular proliferations (benign or malignant). When blood vessels proliferate there may be a palpable component to the skin lesions such as papules, patches, plaques or nodules.

This Albanian patient presented with multiple, asymptomatic, palpable, purple skin lesions on a background of immunosuppression, leading to a clinical diagnosis of Kaposi's sarcoma (KS). This was confirmed histologically by taking a skin biopsy. The histopathology showed the classic spindle cells surrounding slit-like spaces with red blood cells; staining for human herpes virus type 8 (HHV-8) was positive.

This patient's HIV test was negative, and he was therefore diagnosed with disseminated endemic KS. The immunosuppressive medication he was taking for his liver transplant had allowed the proliferation of KS-associated herpes virus (thought to be HHV-8) leading to the development of clinical KS lesions. In the context of transplantation these patients are thought to harbour the latent oncogenic herpes virus, which then reactivates leading to the development of malignant vascular tumours. KS classically affects the skin but mucosal tissue and systemic involvement may also occur. This patient's CT scan was negative for KS lesions in the lung.

So-called iatrogenic KS in liver and renal transplant patients poses a therapeutic challenge. The tumour is chemosensitive and radiosensitive. However, in the context of transplantation, adjustment to the immunosuppressive medication can be highly successful. This patient was switched from tacrolimus to sirolimus (rapamycin) with regression of the tumours. Sirolimus is immunosuppressive and has anti-tumour properties.

Recent evidence from laboratory studies has shown that the tumour is stimulated by iron salts. Transplant recipients often receive multiple blood transfusions leading to possible iron overload, and consequently leave them more susceptible to KS than other iatrogenically immunosuppressed patients.

 KEY POINTS

- Kaposi's sarcoma (KS) is a malignant vascular tumour that occurs in endemic areas, in HIV carriers and organ transplant recipients.
- Immunohistochemical staining for HHV-8 is positive from KS lesions.
- KS in transplant patients can be managed by adjusting the immunosuppressive medication.

History

A 20-year-old man presents to his GP with an intensely pruritic eruption. He is finding that the itching is keeping him awake at night, and consequently it is hard to concentrate in his college exams. He has come to the GP to ask for a sick note. One of his housemates has also recently become itchy and they had begun to suspect their student flat may have an infestation of some sort. He was previously well and takes no regular medication. The patient had applied calamine lotion on the rash as recommended by his local chemist, with little relief.

Examination

There are multiple erythematous papules and excoriations over his limbs and trunk, which are particularly severe over his hands (Fig. 83.1) and on his genital area. There are some very subtle, palpable linear marks running along the sides of his fingers. His scalp, nails and mouth are normal.

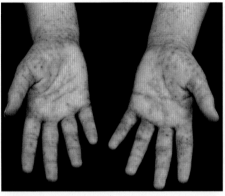

Figure 83.1

Questions

- What is the most likely diagnosis?
- Should the pest control team be requested to visit their flat?
- Who should be treated and with what?

There are few pruritic skin eruptions that keep patients awake at night and usually this is highly suggestive of a scabies infestation. The human mite *Sarcoptes scabiei* is passed from one individual to another, usually by direct skin contact but also through contact with fomites such as bedding and towels. The female parasitic mite that burrows into the skin can only live away from the human host for 1–2 days in the environment. Once the infestation has been transmitted there is a delay of about six weeks before the onset of pruritus, which is a type IV delayed hypersensitivity reaction to the proteins in the mites/eggs/faeces. However, symptoms of pruritus in subsequent infestations can start within days as the individual is already 'primed' to the protein. Several individuals in the same household may be infested simultaneously, especially if living in overcrowded or poor quality accommodation.

Approximately 10 adult females in burrows are present in the human skin during a scabies infestation, and consequently the burrows themselves may be difficult to identify. They are linear wandering lesions, usually most easily seen in the web-spaces of the fingers and on the genitalia. If you look closely with a magnifying lens/dermatoscope

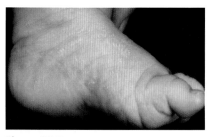

you may just see a small black 'speck' (the mite) at the advancing edge. The remainder of the skin rash consists mainly of erythematous papules and excoriation marks, which reflects a pruritic allergic-type hypersensitivity eruption. Babies have a slightly different clinical presentation in that lesions may look more like blisters and they are particularly common on the soles of the feet (Fig. 83.2) and in the axillae, which should help to distinguish scabies from atopic dermatitis.

Figure 83.2

Crusted scabies occurs in individuals who have thousands of mites in their infestation such that the skin looks as if it has crust or fine scale on the surface. These individuals may be in a poor state of health with a suboptimally functioning immune system.

Infested individuals and all close contacts should be treated with topical permethrin 5% lotion applied to all the skin from the neck downwards (babies should have the face/neck and scalp areas also treated). The treatment should be left on overnight, washed off in the morning and repeated after 7 days as the treatment is not ovicidal. Patients who are immunosuppressed or who have crusted scabies (avoid in children < 5 years old and in pregnancy) can be treated with oral ivermectin 200 μg/kg body weight in 2 doses two weeks apart. Both topical and oral treatments are highly effective. Apparent treatment failures usually result from not all close contacts being treated simultaneously.

The pruritus will continue for approximately 4–6 weeks after successful treatment of the infestation, as this is the time needed for the body to degrade and remove all the mite protein in the skin. Post-scabies treatment therefore consists of soothing anti-itch emollients such as menthol in aqueous cream, and topical steroids can help to alleviate symptoms.

 KEY POINTS

- The pruritus caused by a scabies infestation keeps patients awake at night.
- A detailed history concerning similarly affected household members is helpful in making a diagnosis.
- All close contacts should be treated simultaneously to ensure successful eradication of the mite.

History

A 28-year-old Turkish Cypriot man came to the United Kingdom to visit relatives for a few months. During his visit he noticed that a small erythematous lesion on his nose was increasing in size and his relatives brought him to the accident and emergency department.

He is referred to the dermatology team for an opinion. The lesion is asymptomatic and has been growing slowly over a period of four months. In Cyprus, where he works in the construction industry, he did not recall any history of trauma to the affected area during his work. He does not burn in the sun and is tanned relatively easily. He is otherwise well, and takes no regular medication.

Examination

There is an erythematous nodule at the root of the nose; the overlying epidermis is normal but there is an indurated swelling in the dermis which is firm on palpation (Fig. 84.1). There is no ulceration or evidence of telangiectasia within the lesion. Examination of his mucous membranes is normal, there is no regional lymphadenopathy or organomegaly. He has a BCG vaccination scar on his upper left arm, the rest of his skin check is normal.

🔍 INVESTIGATIONS

A skin biopsy was taken for histology, culture and analysis by polymerase chain reaction (PCR). Full blood count was normal.

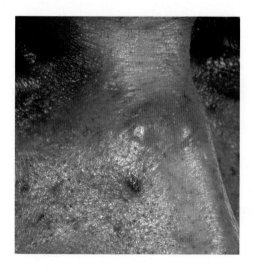

Figure 84.1

Questions

- What is the most likely clinical diagnosis?
- What would you expect the culture and PCR analysis to show?
- How would you manage this patient?

The skin histopathology from the lesion showed ill-defined granulomas with lymphocytes, plasma cells and eosinophils, there was no evidence of vasculitis. Special stains for micro-organisms were negative. The differential diagnoses of cutaneous granulomas include sarcoidosis, tuberculosis, deep fungal infections, leishmaniasis, foreign body reactions, granuloma annulare and granuloma faciale. Microbiological culture from lesional skin grew *Leishmania* protozoan parasites. PCR confirmed the species *Leishmania donovanii* complex. The patient was therefore diagnosed with cutaneous leishmaniasis.

There are many different species of *Leishmania*, each confined to a geographical region of the world and transmitted by the bite of the female sandfly vector. Bites usually occur at night on exposed skin and are not normally painful, therefore patients rarely recall being bitten. Leishmaniasis acquired in Cyprus – so-called 'old world' leishmaniasis – can result in cutaneous or mucocutaneous disease.

At the site of the sandfly bite, classically, a small erythematous non-painful papule forms. Over a few months the lesion increases in size into a nodule that may ulcerate. Localized cutaneous leishmaniasis is usually a self-limiting disease with most lesions healing within 5–15 months. Lesions usually heal with scarring. Treatment aims are to heal lesions more rapidly and try to reduce scarring. In resource-poor settings cryotherapy or heat therapy can be successfully used; however, if available, intra-lesional stibogluconate is highly effective. This pentavalent antimony-containing compound is injected into the lesion at weekly intervals for a few weeks. This patient received five injections over a 6-week period, causing clinical resolution with minimal scarring.

Patients with mucocutaneous or visceral leishmaniasis may be quite unwell with a temperature and malaise. Visceral involvement can lead to a depressed bone marrow (anaemia, leucopenia and thrombocytopenia) and hepatosplenomegaly. Such patients require systemic treatment with intravenous stibogluconate (20–40 days) or intramuscular pentamidine (10 injections given on alternate days) both of which have challenging side-effect profiles. Liposomal amphotericin B (3 mg/kg per day for 5 days plus a further treatment after 1 week) can be effective and is reasonably well tolerated.

 KEY POINTS

- Cutaneous leishmaniasis occurs at the site of a sandfly bite, usually on exposed skin.
- Histopathology and culture from involved skin can confirm the diagnosis; however, PCR is highly specific for species identification.
- Identifying the species of *Leishmania* involved is important as this guides therapy, whether topical or systemic.

History

A 4-year-old boy is referred from the accident and emergency department to the paediatric dermatology clinic, owing to a 1-year history of scaling and crusting of his scalp associated with hair loss. Despite numerous courses of oral antibiotics and topical antifungal creams the eruption had become progressively worse over the last few months. No one else at home is obviously affected. The child is otherwise well.

Examination

The patient is accompanied by his parents and older sibling. There are obvious patches of alopecia over the vertex of his scalp associated with scaling and crusting (Fig. 85.1). The skin is inflamed and erythematous in the affected areas. There is marked occipital lymphadenopathy. The rest of his skin and nails look normal. Examination of his older sibling reveals a diffusely scaly scalp, but no alopecia or lymphadenopathy. The patient's mother is noted to have a scaly annular lesion on her anterior neck, both parents' scalps look normal.

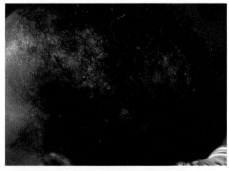

Figure 85.1

INVESTIGATIONS

The whole family had scalp brushings taken for mycological culture. A scraping for mycological microscopy and culture was also taken from the lesion on the mother's neck.

The patient was started on oral therapy daily plus a shampoo, but within five days he had developed a widespread itchy papular rash (Fig. 85.2) and returned to the dermatology clinic.

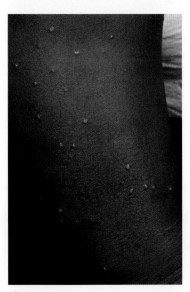

Figure 85.2

Questions

- What disease is affecting the patient's scalp and what is the cause of his widespread rash?
- Which members of the family would you treat and with what agents?
- Is the patient's hair likely to grow back?

This boy presents with a very common scalp complaint of children seen in most urban areas. He is suffering from tinea capitis (scalp 'ringworm') which is a dermatophyte fungal infection. The clinical appearances can be highly variable from marked scaling, crusting, pustules and papules to a frank inflammatory boggy swelling (kerion) with alopecia, to subtle fine diffuse scale only. Children frequently have associated occipital lymphadenopathy.

After starting oral antifungal medication the patient developed a classic pruritic papular 'id' reaction which is an immunological reaction to the infection that can coincide with the start of treatment. It is not an allergy to the antifungal treatment as is frequently assumed. The 'id' reaction can be managed with mild topical steroids and emollients. The oral antifungals should be continued.

The fungus is spread from child to child in schools and between family members at home. Frequently, parents' scalps are spared, however they may develop cutaneous lesions (tinea corporis), especially on their neck and upper trunk where the child's head comes to rest whilst sitting on the parent's lap.

Trichophyton tonsurans is an anthropophilic (human) species, which is most commonly isolated from the mycological culture. The fungal hyphae of *T. tonsurans* penetrate into the hair shaft (endothrix) rendering topical therapy ineffective. Therefore, systemic treatment is required to clear the scalp infection. Screening of family members by taking scalp brushings is recommended as tinea capitis may be very subtle clinically. Mycology cultures can take 6–8 weeks, as the fungus grows slowly; consequently, treatment may need to be started in the first instance on clinical grounds.

Traditionally, children with tinea capitis were treated with oral griseofulvin, however to eradicate *T. tonsurans* high doses are required for up to two months. Oral terbinafine is therefore the treatment of choice in many paediatric dermatology clinics, as it is highly effective and well tolerated. As yet, oral terbinafine is not licensed in children in the UK. Oral terbinafine is given to children daily for 1 month according to their weight: < 20 kg, 62.5 mg; 20–40 kg, 125 mg; > 40 kg, 250 mg. It is good clinical practice to re-brush the scalp after treatment to ensure that there is a mycological as well as clinical cure.

In this case the two children should be treated with oral antifungal medicine and their mother given topical terbinafine 1% cream to treat her tinea corporis. It is a good idea to ask all the family members to use an antifungal shampoo once/twice weekly to reduce the spread of fungus during the treatment course.

Fortunately, the alopecia has a very high chance of complete recovery after treatment, even after a highly inflammatory kerion.

KEY POINTS

- Clinical features of tinea capitis are highly variable, from mild diffuse scale to pustules and swelling.
- Affected children and their close contacts should be screened for tinea capitis by scalp brushings.
- Systemic antifungals should be given, as the majority of cases are caused by endothrix fungi.

History

A 37-year-old healthcare assistant presents to the dermatology clinic with a pruritic eruption over her right knee. The lesion had started as a small erythematous papule and then spread out very gradually to form a scaly, ring-shaped lesion. The itching is not intense but she does find herself scratching. She has no history of previous skin problems. Her 7-year-old son has eczema and a dry scaly scalp. She has used some of her son's cortisone ointment on the lesion, which seemed to reduce the itching and scaling but the lesion has continued to expand.

Examination

There is an annular lesion 9 cm in diameter with a raised edge over the right knee (Fig. 86.1). Marked hyperpigmentation, erythema and multiple papules and pustules are seen at the raised edge. Her scalp and nails are normal, as is the rest of her skin. She has brought her son with her to the clinic; he has a very scaly scalp with patches of alopecia and occipital lymphadenopathy.

INVESTIGATIONS

Mycology scrapings from the edge of the right knee lesion were examined by microscopy (fungal hyphae were seen), and tissue culture (result: *Trichophyton tonsurans*)
Mycology brushings from the son's scalp were examined by tissue culture (result: *T. tonsurans*)

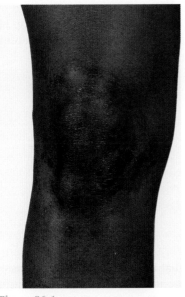

Figure 86.1

Questions

- What is the diagnosis?
- From whom did the patient acquire the infection?
- How would you treat the mother and child?

The healthcare assistant has a cutaneous fungal infection caused by the dermatophyte *Trichophyton tonsurans*. The patient had used a cortisone ointment on the fungal infection which altered the cutaneous appearance. This phenomenon is so-called 'tinea incognito' (steroid-modified tinea), whereby the fungal infection continues to spread outwards but the scale is reduced and small papules and pustules may appear at the growing margin.

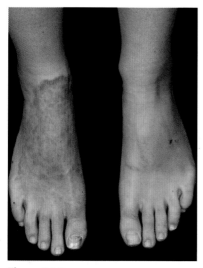

Figure 86.2

T. tonsurans is the main cause of tinea capitis (scalp 'ringworm') in children living in urban areas. The fungus is anthropophilic – that is, passed between humans. The usual cutaneous manifestation of tinea corporis (i.e. not treated with topical corticosteroid) is shown in Figure 86.2. The classic presentation includes annular lesions that are scaly at the edge with central clearing; the eruption is mildly pruritic.

The patient's son had tinea capitis, which is the most likely source of the infection. *T. tonsurans* is likely to spread to adults when the infected child's head comes into direct contact with the adults' skin, usually on the neck / anterior chest where a child's head rests whilst sitting on their lap. If an adult presents with a *T. tonsurans*, ask about contact with children.

Samples for mycology are very easy to take and results are useful in guiding treatment. Skin scrapings can be taken using a blunt scalpel blade from the active edge of the lesions. Samples should be sent to the laboratory in folded coloured paper. Scalp brushings can be taken using plastic sterile disposable travel toothbrushes, using brisk brushing movements back and forth across the scalp. Brush siblings and parents.

!	Clues to the diagnosis of tinea corporis

- *The skin site affected* – fungi often prefer the flexures (groin/axillae)
- *The eruption will often be asymmetrical* – unlike many inflammatory dermatoses such as psoriasis and eczema
- *Concomitant fungal nail infection* – onychomycosis
- *Underlying diseases* – such as diabetes, immunosuppression
- *Others at home are affected* – especially children with tinea capitis
- *Worsening with use of topical steroid*

T. tonsurans is an endothrix fungus, which means that the fungal spores reside inside the hair shaft; consequently, scalp infections need to be managed with systemic antifungal medications. In the past, griseofulvin was used to treat tinea capitis in children at a dose of 10 mg/kg daily for 6–8 weeks, however one month of terbinafine is equally effective and better tolerated at a daily dose depending on the child's weight: < 20 kg, 62.5 mg; 20–40 kg, 125 mg; > 40 kg, 250 mg. Tinea corporis can be managed with topical terbinafine 1% cream used twice daily for 4-6 weeks. Alternatives are oral terbinafine 250 mg daily for 2 weeks or oral itraconazole 400 mg daily for 1 week.

KEY POINTS

- A cutaneous fungal infection should be suspected in a patient with isolated scaly annular lesions.
- Classical signs of tinea can be altered by topical steroid use or secondary bacterial infection.
- Tinea capitis in urban areas is most frequently caused by endothrix fungal species that require systemic therapy.

History

A dermatology opinion is sought for a 47-year-old in-patient on the haematology ward. He has noticed slowly progressive redness and scaling of his feet and left palm, which is minimally itchy. In addition he has extensive discolouration and brittleness of his toenails and fingernails of the left hand. He had first noticed the skin and nail changes 4 months previously. There is no family or personal history of skin/nail problems. He is currently an in-patient, having undergone an autologous stem cell transplantation for multiple myeloma associated with systemic amyloidosis. Prior to the transplant he had been receiving high-dose melphalan.

Examination

The skin on the soles of his feet and left palm is erythematous with scaling and desquamation. Nail plates are dystrophic and brittle distally, Beau's lines are evident (horizontal indentation of the nail plates) and there is associated periungal erythema (Fig. 87.1).

🔍 INVESTIGATIONS

		Normal
White cell count	1.23×10^9/L	$4.00–11.0 \times 10^9$/L
Haemoglobin	9.2 g/dL	11.5–16.5 g/dL
Platelets	38×10^9/L	$150–450 \times 10^9$/L
Neutrophils	0.20×10^9/L	$2.20–6.30 \times 10^9$/L
Lymphocytes	0.98×10^9/L	$1.30–4.00 \times 10^9$/L

Nail clippings and skin scrapings were taken for microscopy and tissue culture.

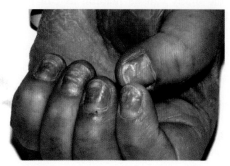

Figure 87.1

Questions

- What is the likely cause of the skin and nail abnormalities?
- What treatment could be offered?

Skin scaling on the hand/foot and nail dystrophy can be associated with palmar–plantar psoriasis, severe pompholyx eczema, or dermatophyte (fungal) infections. As a general rule cutaneous inflammatory disorders are more likely to present in a symmetrical fashion than infections. This patient had been receiving chemotherapy and a stem cell transplantation, and therefore had undergone a prolonged period of immunosuppression, which had left him vulnerable to infections.

Nail clippings and skin scrapings were sent for mycological analysis. Fungal hyphae were seen on microscopy and cultures from skin and nails grew *Trichophyton rubrum*.

Dermatophyte fungi invade the epidermis and keratinized tissues of the skin, nails and hair. Adults are more susceptible than children to tinea pedis (athlete's foot) and onychomycosis (fungal nail infection). It is estimated that about 3–8 per cent of the adult population is affected by onychomycosis. In diabetic patients and those who are immunosuppressed the incidence is higher.

Invasion of the nail plate distally and laterally usually follows chronic tinea pedis. As fungi penetrate through the nail plate it lifts up off the nail bed – so-called onycholysis. The nail plate itself becomes brittle, discoloured and may become hyperkeratotic. The most common fungi implicated in onychomycosis in Europe include *T. rubrum*, *T. interdigitale*, *T. tonsurans* and *Candida albicans*.

Treatment of onychomycosis is guided by the severity, symptoms, number of nails affected, possible drug interactions, drug intolerance and patient expectation. Choosing the right antifungal preparation is aided by the identification of the underlying causative fungus. Dermatophyte fungi including *Trichophyton* spp. can be treated with oral terbinafine (6-12 weeks) or itraconazole (continuous or pulsed for 3–4 months). Topical preparations (applied twice weekly for 6-12 months) are usually reserved for more limited nail disease or for those unable to take oral antifungal drugs.

Candida yeast around the nails is usually present in a mixed infection along with dermatophyte fungi and/or bacteria. Fluconazole orally can be helpful, as can topical clotrimazole, for any associated *Candida* skin involvement.

 KEY POINTS

- Fungal nail infections are most common amongst adults and immunosuppressed patients.
- Onychomycosis causes morbidity and cosmetic embarrassment rather than severe disease.
- Oral antifungal drugs are more effective than topical treatment alone in treating onychomycosis.

History

A 15-year-old girl presents with a 3-month history of hair loss. The girl's mother had noticed an initial small patch of hair loss over the posterior scalp. Her family had thought this might be due to 'stress' as the girl's grandfather had recently died. Subsequently, the initial patch increased in size and over the past six weeks multiple patches of hair loss have been noticed. She has a past history of eczema and hay fever. She is otherwise well and has a family history of hypothyroidism.

Examination

There are multiple patches of alopecia over the occipital and parietal scalp, the skin looks normal (Fig. 88.1). At the periphery of the patches of alopecia are 'exclamation mark' hairs. No erythema or scale is seen on the scalp. The rest of her body hair is normal, as are her nails. There is no occipital lymphadenopathy.

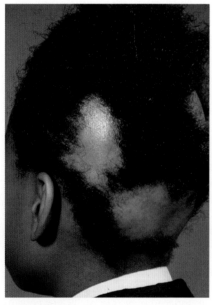

Figure 88.1

Questions

- What is the diagnosis?
- Would you request any investigations?
- How would you manage this patient?

When assessing patients with hair loss it is important to first establish whether the alopecia is focal or diffuse, whether the skin on the scalp is normal or diseased and, if the skin is diseased, is there scarring? This girl had patchy alopecia with normal skin, which is highly suggestive of the diagnosis of alopecia areata. This is an autoimmune disease; inflammatory cells target the growing hairs, which subsequently fall out.

Hair growth is cyclical, with three phases: anagen (growing phase); catagen (resting phase); and telogen (shedding phase). Alopecia areata is a common autoimmune disease that occurs in approximately 1 per cent of the population and generally begins in young adults.

Classically, it presents with well-demarcated circular patches of gradual, asymptomatic hair loss with no evidence of inflammation or scarring over the scalp. Pathognomonic exclamation mark hairs are seen which appear as broken off stubby hairs due to the proximal shaft being narrower than the distal shaft. Eyebrows, eyelashes and the beard area are also affected. Other patterns include totalis where complete hair loss occurs over the entire scalp and universalis where hair is lost from all body sites. In addition, evidence of nail pitting can be seen. The differential diagnosis includes other causes of a non-scarring alopecia including tinea capitis, traction alopecia and trichotillomania (constant rubbing or pulling of the hair).

The course of alopecia areata is unpredictable. Spontaneous remission is common in more patchy disease. When regrowth occurs the hair is much finer and often white or grey initially. After the first episode, 30 per cent of patients regrow the hair within one year. Recurrences are common, however. Poor prognosis is associated with prepubertal onset, occipital involvement, prolonged duration of hair loss in a given area and atopy.

Treatment is dependent on the extent. The prognosis for a solitary, small lesion is excellent, so no treatment may be required as spontaneous regrowth often occurs. For further focal disease, topical or intra-lesional corticosteroids can be helpful. For more extensive disease short courses of systemic corticosteroids, ciclosporin, phototherapy (psoralen–UVA) and topical immunotherapy to induce a contact sensitization with diphencyprone can be useful.

Alopecia areata is associated with other autoimmune diseases including vitiligo, Addison's disease and thyroid disease, which is why the family history of autoimmune disease in this case is relevant. However, studies have shown a concordance rate of 55 per cent in monozygotic twins, suggesting that both genetic and environmental factors are relevant. Atopy also appears to be linked. Therefore, blood tests to rule out other underlying autoimmune diseases should be considered in patients presenting with alopecia areata.

 KEY POINTS

- Hair growth is cyclical, in three phases: anagen, catagen and telogen.
- Alopecia areata can be focal or diffuse.
- 'Exclamation mark' hairs are pathognomonic of alopecia areata.

History

A 55-year-old woman presents with an 18-month history of hair thinning over her frontal scalp. She denies any symptoms from her scalp and has not lost hair elsewhere. She takes hormone replacement therapy and is otherwise well. Her brother and father had both suffered with male pattern baldness in their 40s. Her mother has always had a 'good head of hair'.

Examination

There is diffuse thinning of her hair over the frontal scalp extending to the vertex (Fig. 89.1). The hair that is present is finer in texture and shorter than the hair over the rest of her scalp. The scalp skin appears normal as are her nails.

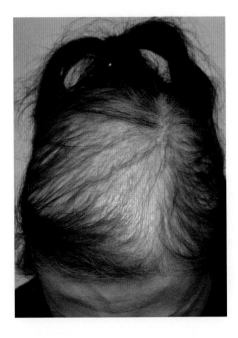

Figure 89.1

Questions

- What is the diagnosis?
- What are the potential treatment options?

This patient is suffering from androgenetic alopecia. She has noticed gradual thinning of her hair, particularly over the frontal scalp and vertex. The family history of hair loss in men is relevant.

Androgenetic alopecia is a very common, progressive hair loss that occurs predominantly in men (male pattern baldness). This occurs due to the combined effect of genetic predisposition and the action of androgens on hair follicles. Dihydrotestosterone (DHT) is believed to shorten the anagen phase (growth phase) causing miniaturization of the hair follicle which then produces finer hairs. The genetic predisposition can be inherited from either parent. In men this can occur at any time after puberty as early as in late teens and is present in 80 per cent by the 7th decade. In women it occurs later and the majority of women will have a normal hormone profile. It is more pronounced after the menopause, most commonly occurring in the 6th decade.

Androgenetic alopecia in men is usually demonstrated by a receding anterior hairline, particularly in the parietal-temporal region resulting in the classical M-shape of hair loss. Following this the vertex (crown) may become affected.

In women the pattern of hair loss is different. They commonly exhibit loss over the frontal scalp and the parietal and temporal regions are spared. If a young woman presents with this pattern of hair loss then she should be examined for signs of virilization such as clitoral hypertrophy, acne and hirsutism. If present, an underlying systemic endocrine disease should be excluded. Testosterone and dehydroepiandrosterone sulphate levels should be measured.

Treatment options include hairpieces such as wigs/weaves and toupées. Topical minoxidil can be effective in some patients in reducing and partially restoring hair loss. Once discontinued though, the effect is lost. Finasteride, which inhibits 5-α-reductase (an enzyme that regulates production of DHT), can slow down hair loss in men. In women who have elevated adrenal androgens, anti-androgen drugs such as spironolactone, cyproterone and cimetidine can be effective. Finally, there may be a role for hair transplantation in some patients.

 KEY POINTS

- Androgenetic alopecia is a common, progressive hair loss occurring predominantly in men.
- Genetic predisposition and the effect of androgens on follicles leads to male pattern baldness.
- In women underlying systemic endocrine disease should be excluded.

History

A 24-year-old woman with type VI skin reports an excess of facial hair and the development of hair over her chest. Her sister and mother are similarly affected, but more mildly. She has become increasingly embarrassed by the problem and consequently has become reclusive. She takes no medication and is systemically well.

Examination

She has increased hair growth over the lateral borders of her face, on her chin and submental regions (Fig. 90.1). Her mid-anterior chest has central dark terminal hairs which extend to the periareolar regions.

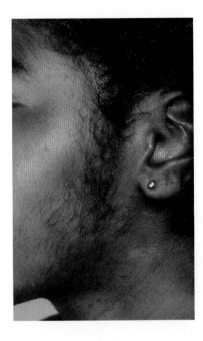

Figure 90.1

Questions

- What is the diagnosis?
- What possible underlying causes need to be excluded?
- How would you manage this patient?

This patient feels she has an excess of facial and body hair, which is referred to as hirsutism. This is a perceived excessive growth of terminal hair in women in a male pattern.

It is a very common problem that occurs predominantly over the upper lip, chin, periareolar regions, abdomen, posterior trunk, shoulders and pubic area. The majority of patients have idiopathic hirsutism. Risk factors include familial and ethnic influences.

Possible underlying causes include ovarian diseases such as polycystic ovarian syndrome and virilizing tumours; adrenal causes, congenital adrenal hyperplasia and Cushing's disease; and iatrogenic cause, androgens and progesterone. In patients presenting with hirsutism it is important to elicit a family and drug history and to look clinically for signs of virilization, which include androgenic alopecia, acne, clitoral hypertrophy and deepening of the voice.

Most patients with hirsutism have a normal menstrual cycle and no signs of virilization. It is therefore unlikely that these patients have a significant endocrine cause. In such patients it is likely that there is increased end-order sensitivity to androgens. Androgens promote conversion of vellus hairs to terminal ones in androgen-sensitive hair follicles (sites such as the chin area.)

Treatment is generally unsatisfactory. Temporary hair removal techniques include waxing, plucking, shaving and threading. More permanent techniques include electrolysis and hair-removal lasers. Anti-androgen therapies include cyproterone acetate, sprinolactone, cimetidine and the oral contraceptive pill.

 KEY POINTS

- Hirsuitism is excessive growth of terminal hair in women in a male pattern.
- It occurs mainly over the upper lip, chin, periareolar regions and pubic area.
- Underlying causes include ovarian diseases and virilizing tumours.

History

A 35-year-old woman presents to the dermatology clinic with several skin lesions over sun-exposed sites. A few lesions on the dorsi of her hands had become slightly tender but are otherwise asymptomatic. More recently she has developed a rapidly growing lesion on her lower lip that bleeds when traumatized. She had undergone cryotherapy and curettage and cautery to several scaly lesions in the past. Twenty years ago she had undergone a renal transplant for renal failure secondary to nephrotic syndrome. She is taking mycophenolate mofetil and azathioprine. When she was a young child she lived in East Africa with her parents who had helped set up a school. She herself had worked with an aid agency based in the United Kingdom. She has no history of atopy and is otherwise well.

Examination

She has a hyperkeratotic cutaneous horn on her lower lip (Fig. 91.1) with multiple erythematous scaly patches over the dorsum of the hands, forearms and face. In addition there are several previous surgical scar sites.

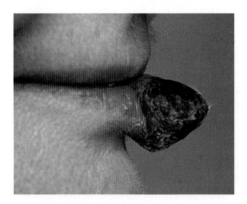

Figure 91.1

Questions

- What is the most likely diagnosis?
- What dermatological advice should be given to transplant recipients?

Immunosuppressed patients are more vulnerable to the damaging effects of high-intensity ultraviolet (UV) light than immunocompetent ones. The most likely diagnosis in this case is a squamous cell carcinoma (SCC) on the lip, multiple actinic keratoses and superficial basal cell carcinomas (BCCs) elsewhere. Multiple skin cancers have arisen in this patient due to a combination of factors including immunosuppressant medication, fair skin and significant sun exposure in childhood.

Skin malignancy is the most frequently reported cancer in organ transplant recipients: the prevalence is 16.5 per cent in the UK. The majority of these are non-melanoma skin cancers (NMSCs) such as SCCs and BCCs. A NMSC presents at an earlier age and spreads more rapidly in transplant recipients than in the general population. Patients frequently have multiple lesions over time and consequently suffer substantial morbidity and a seven-fold increase in mortality from skin cancer. There is also an increased risk of developing malignant melanoma and Kaposi's sarcoma. In addition premalignant lesions are very commonly seen including actinic keratoses and Bowen's disease.

UV radiation is a significant risk factor for the development of skin malignancy. Organ transplant recipients require life-long immunosuppressant medication to prevent host organ rejection. The immunosuppressants impair the capacity of immune surveillance to repair and destroy UV damage and therefore leave patients vulnerable to skin cancers. In addition, transplant recipients are susceptible to infection with human papilloma virus, which may be associated with the development of some SCCs.

Photoprotection post-transplantation is essential in these patients. The high incidence, rapid growth, and increased metastatic potential of skin malignancy in these patients justifies the surveillance service provided in many dermatology units. In order to reduce the tumour burden in these patients, their management requires an interdisciplinary approach. Early detection and appropriate treatment of lesions are essential.

Complete excision is the 'gold standard' for SCCs in transplant recipients, if possible. Treatments of premalignant lesions may include topical therapy with 5-fluorouracil, 5% imiquimod cream, cryotherapy, and curettage and cautery. Finally, those transplant recipients who have had multiple SCCs should be commenced on a life-long oral retinoid such as acitretin to help reduce the number of new skin cancers developing.

 KEY POINTS

- Skin cancer is the most frequently reported cancer in organ transplant recipients.
- The majority of these are non-melanoma skin cancers such as SCCs and BCCs.
- Photoprotection post-transplantation is essential in these patients.

History

A 37-year-old man presents with a rash and diarrhoea to the haematology out-patient team. Six months previously he had developed red patches on his skin, which then became pale and gradually felt firm and tight. He describes stiffness of his elbow and knee joints, such that he is having trouble straightening his limbs. One year previously he had undergone a matched, unrelated, allogenic bone marrow transplant for acute myeloid leukaemia. He is taking multiple medications including aciclovir, co-trimoxazole, penicillin V, itraconazole and omeprazole.

Examination

He has extensive skin changes over his trunk and limbs with erythematous patches with hypopigmented centres (Fig. 92.1). There is mottled hyperpigmentation and generalized thickening of the skin, which appears waxy and feels tight. Also, fixed flexion deformities are present over his elbows and knees.

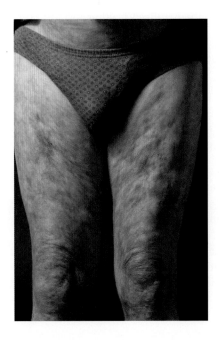

Figure 92.1

Questions

- What is the diagnosis?
- What other systems can be involved?
- How would you manage this patient?

This patient was diagnosed with chronic graft-versus-host disease (GVHD). Skin changes characterized by thickening and tightening after bone marrow transplantation are referred to as sclerodermoid GVHD.

GVHD is an immune disorder that commonly follows bone marrow transplantation. It is less common after solid organ transplantation and, rarely, has also been reported in patients after blood transfusion and by maternal–fetal transfusion. GVHD results from a reaction of incompatible, immunocompetent donor cells against the tissue of an immunocompetent host. Acute and chronic disease are described both of which increase the patient's susceptibility to infection.

Chronic GVHD is said to occur more than 100 days after transplantation. Patients may have had acute GVHD (usually between 14 and 21 days post-transplantation) or it arises de novo. Cutaneous disease has different morphological types. These include lichenoid, sclerodermoid and eczematous types. Lichenoid disease is characterized by flat-topped violaceous 'lichen–planus'-like papules and plaques, which manifest initially on the extremities but can become generalized. Mucosal disease is also seen. Sclerodermoid disease occurs predominantly over the trunk and upper lower limbs and the skin is described as 'hardening' or 'tight'. This disease can also become generalized leading to joint contractures. Hair loss is also a common feature, which is usually permanent.

GVHD may also affect the eyes, mouth, joints, gastrointestinal tract (diarrhoea), liver (transaminitis) and respiratory system.

Prevention of GVHD is the mainstay of treatment. Chronic GVHD carries a high morbidity and mortality. It is commonly associated with recurrent and occasionally fatal bacterial infections, which are the main cause of death in patients with GVHD. Patients are immunosuppressed with a variety of medication including ciclosporin, mycophenolate and tacrolimus with or without prednisone.

Managing skin GVHD is dependent on the extent and affected site. For limited disease topical therapy with potent corticosteroids can be of benefit. For more extensive disease the aim is to treat GVHD before life-threatening sepsis occurs. High-dose systemic corticosteroids are usually added to the immunosuppressant regime. Phototherapy with psoralen–UVA and high-dose long-wave ultraviolet (UV) radiation (UVA1) may reduce the severity of the cutaneous skin problems. In addition, to reduce the amount of immunosuppression required, extracorporeal photophoresis can be effective.

 KEY POINTS

- Graft-versus-host disease (GVHD) is an immune disorder that may occur after bone marrow transplantation.
- Acute and chronic forms of GVDH have been described.
- Different types of cutaneous GVHD include lichenoid, sclerodermoid and eczematous.

History

A 22-month-old girl is referred with a persistent colour change in a patchy distribution over her body. She is otherwise well and fully vaccinated to date. She was born post-term at 41 weeks' gestation by normal vaginal delivery. Her mother reports that she had a blistering skin rash at birth and a 'high white cell count'. She was treated with antibiotics for one week on the neonatal unit and had extensive tests to rule out viral illness, all of which were negative. Her mother shares neonatal photos and is certain that the areas of colour change do not correspond with the areas of previous blistering.

Her family history is remarkable in that her maternal grandmother recalls her mother suffering from a similar transient neonatal blistering eruption. She has an older sister aged 7 years and her mother has been investigated for recurrent miscarriages.

Examination

The girl is clearly thriving with height and weight between the 75th and 91st centiles for her age. She has achieved age-appropriate developmental milestones. She has striking linear streaked and whorled areas of brown hyperpigmentation, predominantly over her trunk but also involving her legs. Figure 93.1 shows a well-defined, irregular linear streak of hyperpigmentation extending along the dorsal aspect of her left leg. The distribution of the colour changes corresponds with Blaschko's lines. She has marked ridging of three fingernails and one toenail. All twenty of her deciduous teeth have erupted; she has two peg-shaped teeth. Her mother is also happy to be examined and she has subtle skin changes composed of fine pale, hairless, atrophic, 'porcelain'-like streaks over her posterior calves. She has two hypoplastic nails and one conical tooth.

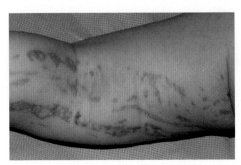

Figure 93.1

Questions

- What is the diagnosis?
- What is the implication of this diagnosis?
- What is the explanation for the distribution of the hyperpigmentation?

This is the classical clinical scenario of an uncommon genodermatosis called incontinentia pigmenti (IP). Skin features are subdivided into four stages: vesicular, verrucous, hyperpigmented, and atrophic. There are various hair, nail, dental, ophthalmological and neurological anomalies described in association with IP. The differential diagnosis of the neonatal vesicular stage, which is typically associated with a peripheral eosinophilia, includes infections (bullous impetigo, herpes simplex, varicella), Langerhans cell histiocytosis, epidermolysis bullosa, bullous mastocytosis and autoimmune blistering diseases.

IP is an X-linked dominant disorder, lethal in the majority of males *in utero*, explaining the mother's recurrent miscarriages. The pathogenic mutation occurs within the *NEMO/IKK γ* gene. Genetic testing is available, although prenatal testing is not generally offered as prognosis for affected females is generally excellent and affected male fetuses do not generally survive into the second trimester.

Clinical presentations vary, even among family members (Table 93.1). The differences in clinical phenotype expression are attributed to lyonization resulting in functional mosaicism, which in the skin manifests along the curvilinear lines of Blaschko. These represent random X-inactivation and migration of clonal epidermal cells along embryological developmental lines. Cells expressing the mutated X chromosome selectively eliminate, and affected females have an extremely skewed X-inactivation pattern.

Table 93.1 **Features of the cutaneous stages of IP**

Stage	Range	Features
1	Birth to 20 weeks approx.	Erythema, vesicles in linear distribution on torso and/or extremities
2	4 weeks to 6 months	Verrucous hyperkeratotic plaques and papules, mainly over extremities
3	20 weeks to puberty approx.	Streaks and whorls of brown/grey pigmentation following Blaschko's lines, mainly on trunk
4	Early teens to adulthood	Pale, hairless and atrophic streaks, mainly on extremities

KEY POINTS

- Incontinentia pigmenti (IP) is an uncommon genodermatosis with effects on the neuroectoderm.
- IP is an X-linked dominant disease, lethal to affected males *in utero*.
- Clinical features vary according to the random inactivation of the affected X chromosome and vary with age.

History

A 17-year-old woman is brought to the accident and emergency department by ambulance. She had collapsed in the high street; witnesses called an ambulance immediately as she began to fit. She had two further fits on the way to hospital and the paramedical team described classic generalized tonic–clonic seizures, including a stereotypical ictal cry. She is drowsy and confused on arrival. Her Medi-Alert bracelet confirms that she is known to have epilepsy and that she has another diagnosis, 'XP'. Her family are on their way to the hospital. In the meantime the medical team ensures that she is now stable.

Examination

She appears to be in a deep sleep and is difficult to rouse, although she withdraws from pain. Her blood pressure is 105/60 mmHg, heart rate 68 beats/min and respiratory rate 12 breaths/min. She is clearly still in a post-ictal state. There are marked skin changes affecting all exposed areas of skin, particularly her face (especially cheeks, nose and pinna of her ears), neck, 'V' of the chest and the dorsa of her hands, but not affecting her trunk or other clothed areas. There is poikiloderma (skin atrophy, and telangiectasias with mottled hyperpigmentation and hypopigmentation) (Fig. 94.1). She has bilateral ectropions and a narrow 'pinched' nose.

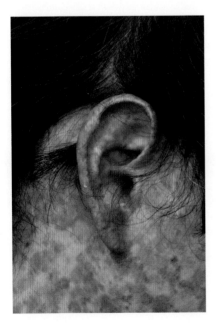

Figure 94.1

Questions

- The distribution of the skin changes suggests a role for what environmental factor?
- What is XP?
- What skin complications can occur in XP?

The distribution of this patient's skin changes is typical for a photodermatosis, occurring on sites most exposed to direct sunlight. Areas more protected from sunlight – such as the scalp, upper eyelids, infranasal and submental areas, as well as fully clothed areas – are typically spared. The changes described are chronic and this is likely to represent a longstanding condition. The most common causes for photosensitive eruptions include drug reactions; however, although neuroleptic medications such as phenothiazines may be implicated, anti-epileptic medications are not particularly associated with phototoxic eruptions except in the context of porphyria. The only porphyria with prominent chronic cutaneous findings is porphyria cutanea tarda (PCT) (acute photosensitivity is seen in other cutaneous porphyrias). PCT is characterized by skin fragility with tense haemorrhagic vesicles and bullae over sun-exposed sites, with hypertrichosis, atrophy and milia developing.

XP stands for xeroderma pigmentosum, a rare autosomal recessive disorder characterized by a cellular hypersensitivity to ultraviolet (UV) radiation resulting from a defect in DNA repair. Individuals with XP develop multiple cutaneous neoplasms at a young age (from 4 to 5 years of age). All forms of skin cancer are described in XP, including basal cell carcinomas, squamous cell carcinomas and malignant melanoma. They are more prevalent over sun-exposed skin, but can also affect the eyes and even buccal mucosa. Neurological problems, including epilepsy, ataxia, spasticity or developmental delay, are present in approximately 20 per cent of patients with XP.

The goals of treatment of patients with XP are to minimize morbidity and prevent mortality primarily through sun protection, through use of sunscreens and sun avoidance measures. Regular skin surveillance, as well as ophthamological and neurological review, are part of routine care of patients with XP.

 KEY POINTS

- Xeroderma pigmentosa (XP) is a rare autosomal recessive skin disorder characterized by dramatic and early-onset photodamage of sun-exposed areas of the skin.
- XP is caused by an inherited defect in repair of UV-induced DNA damage.
- Skin cancers arise from a young age, are typically multiple and result in significant morbidity and potentially early death.

History

A 28-year-old man attends your clinic with his girlfriend. He has had dry skin since birth, although it has been worse since he became a teenager. His skin is generally itchy and requires regular application of emollients and vigorous twice-weekly exfoliation while washing. He is otherwise fit and healthy and a well-adjusted individual. He is planning to get married and would like information about the risk of his children being affected with the same skin condition. He knows other family members who are similarly affected. There is no history of consanguinity. He reports that all affected children were born by emergency caesarean section after very long labour (Fig. 95.1).

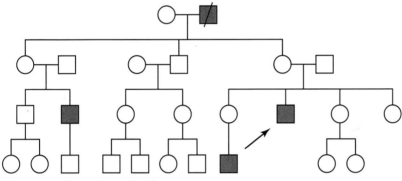

Figure 95.1 The patient's family tree.

Examination

On examination he has normal teeth, hair and nails. He has generally dry skin with prominent adherent grey-brown scales over the extensor surfaces of his neck and limbs (Fig. 95.2). He has adherent bran-like scale throughout his scalp. There is no erythroderma or blistering. His hands and feet are almost unaffected, with little scale and no hyperlinearity or keratoderma.

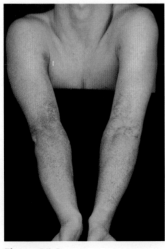

Figure 95.2

Questions

- What is the diagnosis and pattern of inheritance?
- How would you advise this couple about risk to a future generation?

ANSWER 95

This case is a presentation of X-linked ichthyosis. In this condition dryness and scaliness of the skin is often present from birth, and gradually becomes more prominent in late childhood. The build-up of adherent scale imparts a 'dirty appearance' to the skin. Typically, the ichthyosis involves particularly the posterior neck, upper trunk, and extensor surfaces of the extremities, with sparing of the flexures as well as palms and soles (palmoplantar hyperlinearity is a feature of ichthyosis vulgaris). It is one of the most frequent enzyme disorders in humans with an incidence of approximately 1 in 6000 males. It is due to a deficiency of steroid sulphatase (STS), which leads to epidermal barrier defect and corneocyte (or essentially scale) retention.

Most affected individuals regard it as an annoyance, although it can be emotionally challenging in childhood and adolescence. Cryptorchidism can be associated in up to 20 per cent of cases. STS deficiency slows the delivery of an infant because of insufficient cervical dilatation. A relative failure occurs in the response to intravenous oxytocin. Since both are indications for caesarean delivery or forceps delivery, an increased perinatal morbidity and mortality may occur.

Other differential diagnoses to consider include ichthyosis vulgaris (associated with palmar hyperlinearity, atopy and an autosomal dominant inheritance pattern) and lamellar ichthyosis (autosomal recessive inheritance). The diagnosis of X-linked ichthyosis can be confirmed by biochemical assay of STS and by genetic testing.

You can reassure the patient that his sons will not be affected, however his daughters will be obligate carriers. His extended family would benefit from genetic counselling and advice. In particular his female relatives should inform obstetric teams about the possible complications related to prolonged labour or delayed delivery.

 KEY POINTS

- X-linked ichthyosis is caused by steroid sulphatase deficiency.
- The condition is managed with emollients, keratolytics and mechanical exfoliation, with most patients considering it to be an annoyance without significant morbidity.
- It is associated with prolonged labour and, less commonly, cryptorchidism.

History

A 14-year-old boy attends the dermatology out-patient clinic with his mother. He is increasingly troubled by blisters. The blisters affect the plantar surfaces of his feet, particularly the heel, below the metatarsal heads and toes. They have also occurred on his fingers following an exam last year, and a recent school ski-trip provoked blisters over his shins. The appearance of blisters on his feet is directly related to activity and they occur with relatively less activity in summer.

He is otherwise well and not on medication. His mother and one of his two older sisters also suffer with blisters. They have only experienced plantar blisters, and comment that new shoes or walking further than 1.6 km can provoke blisters. They limit their activity and the types of footwear accordingly. None of the family was affected with blisters at birth.

Examination

There is nothing abnormal to find on full examination except for several tense non-inflammatory blisters in an asymmetrical distribution over the weight-bearing aspects of the plantar surface of both feet (Fig. 96.1). He has no skin lesions elsewhere.

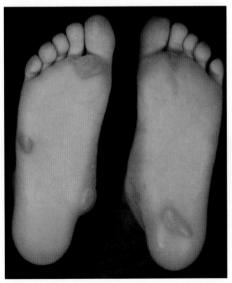

Figure 96.1

Questions

- What is the diagnosis?
- What investigations can you perform to confirm the diagnosis?
- How would you manage this patient?

The patient gives a story which is suggestive of a mechano-bullous skin disorder (blisters due to skin fragility occurring at sites of friction). The positive family history supports an autosomal dominant pattern of inheritance. Apparent onset around adolescence is not unusual and often relates to growth, weight gain and increased physical activity. This patient's history is typical of epidermolysis bullosa (EB) simplex with a localized distribution (also referred to as Webber–Cockayne syndrome).

EB simplex is a group of disorders characterized by intra-epidermal blistering. The disease phenotype can range from mild to severe. The mildest and most common form is EB simplex localized. Although it can present in infancy or childhood, presentation in adulthood or even non-presentation (such as the patient's mother and sister) is not uncommon. Blistering is worse in warm weather as sweat increases friction in footwear.

Biopsy of affected skin is not performed, as the plantar surface of the feet heals poorly. Gently rubbing an unaffected area of non-plantar skin for a biopsy can produce a subclinical blister which will demonstrate the ultrastructural basis of skin fragility. Demonstration of a pathogenic mutation within *Keratin5* or *Keratin14* will confirm the diagnosis.

The management of EB simplex is:

1. avoidance of new blisters by reducing sweat and minimizing friction within footwear, as well as practical and supportive advice around school, work and leisure activities;
2. 'popping' blisters using aseptic methods to relieve pressure and pain and prevention of infection within blisters and erosions, with special dressings which can be removed without trauma to the skin;
3. treatment of callosities which form around areas of frequent blistering, but can act as foci for the development of new blisters;
4. offering adequate and targeted pain control for episodes of blisters as well as chronic neuropathic pain; and
5. genetic counselling.

 KEY POINTS

- There are different forms of epidermolysis bullosa with site and severity of blistering varying according to the molecular defect.
- EB simplex localized is due to dominant negative mutation of either *Keratin 5* or *14* (autosomal dominant pattern of inheritance).
- Practical advice around reducing blistering, blister management and pain control are the cornerstones of management.

History

A 9-year-old boy attends the paediatric dermatology clinic. Both he and his parents are concerned about an accumulation of facial lesions over several months. His mother has tried several over-the-counter anti-acne remedies without apparent benefit. He is otherwise well, although in comparison with his siblings (two older sisters) he has struggled at school; closer questioning suggests that he has problems academically as well as with his behaviour, although this has never been formally evaluated. He does not take medication. His family are all well, his parents are non-consanguineous.

Examination

He has symmetrically distributed red to pink papules, each measuring 1–3 mm in diameter localized to the nasolabial folds and extending to cheeks, nostrils and also the chin (Fig. 97.1). The individual lesions are smooth and firm. Examination of his skin under Wood's light demonstrates six hypomelanotic macules over his lower back, abdomen and buttocks. Examination of his cardiorespiratory system reveals a midsystolic ejection murmur. His neurological system is normal including fundoscopy, vision and hearing. He does appear to be easily frustrated and requires significant reassurance from his mother throughout the examination, avoiding eye contact and following only the instructions of his mother. His abdomen is soft and there are no palpable masses.

Both of his parents also agreed to full skin examination and no abnormalities were detected.

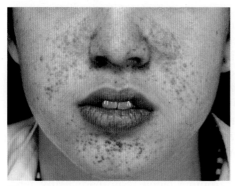

Figure 97.1

Questions

- What are these lesions?
- With what are they associated?
- How would you investigate further?

These lesions are facial angiofibromas (formerly also called adenoma sebaceum). These lesions, associated with hypomelanotic 'ash-leaf' macules, are features of tuberous sclerosis complex. Other cutaneous features include shagreen patch, fibrous plaques, periungual fibromas and confetti-like hypopigmentation. Autosomal dominantly inherited mutations of two genes, *TSC1* (chromosomal locus, 9q34; gene product hamartin) and *TSC2* (16p13; tuberin), can cause tuberous sclerosis complex, which has a broad clinical spectrum. There is a high rate of de-novo mutations with 50–70 per cent of cases presenting as such. Promising new systemic treatments known as mTOR inhibitors are being trialled for complications of tuberous sclerosis. Examination of family members, however, can detect features of a less severe phenotype.

Diagnosis is based on a constellation of clinical features. Definite tuberous sclerosis complex is diagnosed by the presence of either two major features, or one major feature plus two minor features. Presentation with fewer features may fall into categories of probable or possible tuberous sclerosis. A thorough skin examination is important, as skin signs are identified in the majority of affected individuals. Ash-leaf hypomelanotic macules may be present from birth or infancy. Shagreen patches or facial plaques often appear during the first decade. Facial angiofibromas commonly develop in late childhood or around puberty, often stabilizing at puberty. Periungual fibromas often begin at puberty and may continue to accumulate with age.

The clinical scenario presents four issues that need to be addressed: (1) question mark over neurodevelopment; (2) possible pathological cardiac murmur; (3) potential for other occult hamartomas; and (4) implications for other family members.

1. Further investigation of neurodevelopment would include a multiprofessional assessment, ideally within a Child Development Centre, by a community paediatrician, an educational psychologist and a speech therapist. Over 50 per cent of individuals with tuberous sclerosis complex have a low intelligence quotient (IQ) or developmental disorder (particularly autism or language disorders). Unrecognized petit mal seizures can cause problems with school performance, justifying an assessment by a paediatric neurologist with or without electroencephalographic monitoring. A CT scan of the brain would look for evidence of subependymal nodules which may be calcified; MRI is more sensitive in the detection of subependymal giant cell astrocytomas.

2. Further assessment of the cardiac murmur would entail an ECG and echocardiogram to detect cardiac rhabdomyomas. These lesions usually regress with age and are not treated unless of functional significance.

3. Other baseline investigations would include routine blood tests (particularly renal function), renal ultrasound scan, and ophthalmology review (looking for translucent retinal nodules which may represent hamartomas or astrocytomas). Dental pits may also be found.

4. Family members should be offered renal biochemistry and ultrasonography as well as fundoscopy. Even in cases of apparent de-novo mutation unaffected parents of children with tuberous sclerosis complex have a recurrence risk of 1–2 per cent in subsequent pregnancies. Genetic counselling should be initiated.

Characteristic features of tuberous sclerosis complex

Major features
- Intracranial tumours: cortical tubers, subependymal nodules, subependymal giant cell astrocytomas
- Skin lesions: three or more hypomelanotic ash-leaf spots (Fig. 97.2), facial angiofibromas or forehead plaques, shagreen patches (Fig 97.2), ungual or periungual fibromas in the absence of trauma
- Cardiac rhabdomyomas
- Lymphangioleiomyomatosis, renal angiomyolipomas
- Retinal hamartomas

Minor features
- Mouth: dental pits, gingival fibromas
- Confetti skin lesions, bone cysts
- Hamartomatous rectal polyps, multiple renal cysts
- Other nonrenal hamartomas
- Achromic lesions of the retina
- Radial migration lines of cerebral white matter

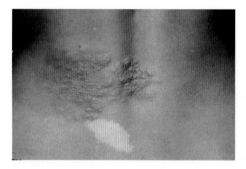

Figure 97.2

 KEY POINTS

- Tuberous sclerosis complex is one of the most common neurocutaneous disorders.
- The disease has a broad clinical spectrum affecting almost all organ systems.
- It is due to an autosomal dominant mutation in one of two tumour suppressor genes encoding the proteins tuberin and hamartin.

History

A 68-year-old woman presents with a 3-week history of worsening back pain. She has been feeling tired for three months and is also complaining of gradually progressive tongue 'thickening'. She is otherwise well and has not attended her GP for more than five years. She is on no medication.

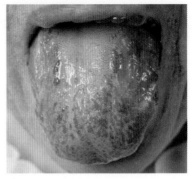

Examination

She is pale and has marked tenderness on palpation of specific areas over her lumbar spine. She has an enlarged tongue, with a smooth papulo-nodular pink infiltrate disrupting the papillae (Fig. 98.1). There is similar involvement of the mucosal aspect of the

Figure 98.1

upper lip extending onto the vermillion lip. Examination of her cardiorespiratory and abdominal systems is normal. She has no palpable lymphadenopathy.

INVESTIGATIONS		
Haemoglobin	9.7 g/dL	13.3–17.7 g/dL
Mean corpuscular volume	77 fL	80–99 fL
White cell count	4.1×10^9/L	$3.9–10.6 \times 10^9$/L
Platelets	138×10^9/L	$150–440 \times 10^9$/L
Erythrocyte sedimentation rate	103 mm/h	< 10 mm/h
Sodium	136 mmol/L	135–145 mmol/L
Potassium	4.1 mmol/L	3.5–5.0 mmol/L
Urea	5.3 mmol/L	2.5–6.7 mmol/L
Creatinine	72 μmol/L	70–120 μmol/L
Albumin	38 g/L	35–50 g/L
Bilirubin	12 mmol/L	3–17 mmol/L
Alanine transaminase	17 IU/L	5–35 IU/L
Alkaline phosphatase	186 IU/L	30–300 IU/L
Urine dipstick	++ protein	
Blood film	Microcytic, normochromic anaemia	

Questions

- What is the likely unifying diagnosis?
- What is occurring in the patient's mouth?

The likely unifying diagnosis in an elderly patient presenting with back pain, anaemia, elevated ESR and an infiltrative process involving the tongue and proteinuria is multiple myeloma, a disease characterized by malignant proliferation of plasma cells and consequent abundance of a monoclonal paraprotein. The presentation of myeloma can be highly variable. The diagnosis can be confirmed by demonstration of a plasma cell clone within the bone marrow and a paraprotein within blood and/or urine. Hypercalcaemia is a common complication.

The infiltration of her tongue and mucosal lip is due to the deposition of light-chain amyloid (AL). Amyloid is defined as in-vivo deposited material distinguished by fibrillar electron micrographic appearance. All types of amyloid consist of a major fibrillar protein that defines the type of amyloid, which can be classified as systemic, hereditary, localized, or organ specific. Cutaneous involvement can occur as an isolated phenomenon or as a manifestation of systemic disease. Mucocutaneous lesions are common in systemic AL and include waxy nodules and plaques, ecchymoses, pinch purpuras, sclerodermoid skin changes and haemorrhagic bullae.

Careful examination and investigation for other systemic amyloid involvement is required. Typical extracutaneous sites include heart, kidney, peripheral nerve, gastrointestinal tract, and respiratory tract. Although patients with both myeloma and systemic amyloidosis associated with other diseases can benefit in terms of symptom control from treatment, there is currently no cure for either condition.

 KEY POINTS

- Multiple myeloma can have a highly variable presentation and potential complications include deposition of light-chain systemic amyloid.
- AL amyloidosis can have a variable presentation, but should prompt investigation particularly for an underlying plasma cell dyscrasia.
- There is no curative treatment for AL amyloidosis.

History

A 59-year-old woman presents with a gradually worsening eruption over 7 weeks. The eruption is pruritic and has not responded to the application of emollients and moderately potent topical glucocorticoids. She has no previous history of skin lesions and reports that she is otherwise well, although she has a poor appetite and has lost 8 kg body weight over the past three months. She does not take medication. She works as a shop assistant and consumes 10 units of alcohol per week. She stopped smoking four years ago.

Examination

The patient's pulse is 76/min and blood pressure 128/76 mmHg. Her striking skin eruption involves the trunk, limbs and neck. There are widespread macular erythematous bands with a wood-grain–like and whorled concentric configuration and fine scaling along the borders (Fig. 99.1). There are no abnormalities on examination of her cardiovascular and respiratory systems. Her abdomen is soft and non-tender with no masses palpable. She has no breast masses. She has a firm 1.5 × 2.0-cm left supraclavicular lymph node.

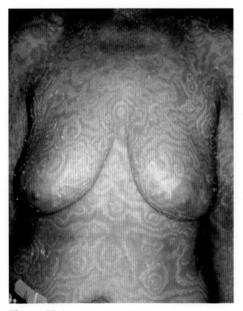

Figure 99.1

		Normal
Haemoglobin	10.3 g/dL	13.3–17.7 g/dL
Mean corpuscular volume	75 fL	80–99 fL
White cell count	3.7 × 10⁹/L	3.9–10.6 × 10⁹/L
Platelets	253 × 10⁹/L	150–440 × 10⁹/L
Blood film:	Hypochromic microcytic anaemia	
Sodium	136 mmol/L	135–145 mmol/L
Potassium	4.6 mmol/L	3.5–5.0 mmol/L
Urea	7.3 mmol/L	2.5–6.7 mmol/L
Creatinine	123 µmol/L	70–120 µmol/L
Albumin	30 g/L	35–50 g/L
Glucose	4.6 mmol/L	4.0–6.0 mmol/L
Bilirubin	12 µmol/L	3–17 µmol/L
Alanine transaminase	63 IU/L	5–35 IU/L
Alkaline phosphatase	865 IU/L	30–300 IU/L
CEA (cancer embryonic antigen)	23 ng/mL	< 2.5 ng/mL
CA 125	26 U/mL	< 35 U/mL (post-menopause)
Tests for ENA, ANA and ANCA (antibodies)	All negative	
Fine needle aspiration (FNA) of palpable lymph node	Smear demonstrates lymph node infiltration by cells of adenocarcinoma morphology	

Questions
- What is this eruption?
- Is there a differential diagnosis?
- What further investigations would you perform?
- What is the management of this patient?

The very striking appearance of this eruption is pathognomonic of erythema gyratum repens (EGR) and potentially a paraneoplastic process. Approximately 80 per cent of patients with EGR have an underlying malignancy. It can also be associated with connective tissue disease (CREST, systemic lupus erythematosus) or infection (such as tuberculosis). The characteristic concentric erythematous bands forming a wood-grain appearance help distinguish EGR from other figurate erythemas, such as erythema annulare centrifugum (may also be paraneoplastic or associated with drugs or other systemic illnesses), erythema migrans (associated with Lyme disease), and erythema marginatum rheumaticum (occurring in association with rheumatic fever). EGR does not respond to skin targeted therapy but rather to treatments aimed at underlying disease.

This clinical picture is highly suggestive of an underlying malignancy. The palpable left supraclavicular lymph node (Virchow's node) with FNA findings of adenocarcinoma points towards gastric pathology.

The next investigations for this patient are an oesophago-gastro-doudenoscopy (OGD) and CT scans of the chest and abdomen. These investigations demonstrated a polypoid gastric adenocarcinoma with lymph node involvement. Resection of the malignancy and lymph node dissection resulted in rapid resolution of the skin eruption.

The differential diagnosis of figurate erythemas

- Dermatophyte infections – usually associated with superficial scale, which contains spores or hyphae, visible on direct microscopy and will culture on appropriate medium
- Annular urticaria – often occurs with more characteristic lesions of urticaria elsewhere, symptoms of pruritus, transient lesions
- Annular psoriasis – unstable psoriasis (e.g. pustular psoriasis) may have an annular configuration
- Subacute lupus erythematosus – often over photo-exposed sites but may be generalized, check Ro/La as well as other lupus-associated autoantibodies
- Bullous pemphigoid – early (prebullous) lesions are intensely pruritic and urticated, may be annular
- Erythema multiforme – typically targetoid lesions, usually acral ± mucosal. Early lesions may be annular before dusky necrosis of central lesion develops
- Necrolytic migratory erythema – rare annular eruption affecting peri-oral, genital and acral skin, erosive or bullous annular lesions, associated with underlying glucagonoma (closely resembles acrodermatitis enteropathica of infancy)
- Erythema gyratum repens
- Erythema annulare centrifugum
- Erythema migrans

 KEY POINTS

- The striking configuration of the erythema is pathognomonic of erythema gyratum repens (EGR).
- EGR is frequently a paraneoplastic process.
- Patients presenting with this eruption should be investigated for underlying systemic disease and in particular malignancy.

History

The teachers of an 11-year-old girl, who has just started a new school, ask her parents to bring her to your attention. They are concerned that the scarring on her legs might be non-accidental. Her mother doesn't hesitate to attend for a medical opinion and presents the next day.

The child is the youngest of four siblings. She was born at 36 weeks' gestation following premature rupture of membranes. She required an inguinal hernia repair at the age of 18 months. Of note, she has had two injuries that were difficult to explain. When 26 months old she dislocated her shoulder during 'boisterous' play with her father and older sisters, and at the age of 5 years she required plastic surgical intervention to a laceration at her left elbow following a relatively minor fall, and despite sutures the wound dehisced and healed poorly. At the age of 3 years she was also investigated at her mother's request for easy bruising, but all blood tests were normal. She has required podiatric attention because of pain in her ankles and feet, which has been attributed to 'flat feet', and she uses orthotic supports in her footwear. Her mother also comments that the child is noticeably more easily fatigued than her siblings and, tellingly, also mentions that she is 'double-jointed'.

Examination

There are multiple loose, atrophic scars over her knees and shins (Fig. 100.1). Her surgical scars have a similar 'cigarette paper', distended appearance. Her skin in general feels very soft, smooth and 'doughy'. It recoils promptly after stretching. She has a Beighton score of 9 (maximum score). The remainder of her physical examination, including eyes, teeth and cardiovascular system, is normal. Her mother's physical examination is unremarkable.

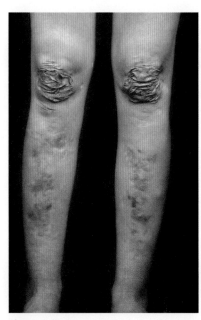

Figure 100.1

Questions

- What differential diagnoses should be considered?
- What is the relevance of the Beighton score?
- What is the management of this patient?

The important features are skin fragility (explaining the easy bruising, multiplicity of scars and need for plastic surgery intervention), abnormal scarring (wound dehiscence and atrophic scars) and hypermobile joints (explaining fatiguability, joint dislocations and high Beighton score). Non-accidental injury is frequently considered before the correct diagnosis is reached. Epidermolysis bullosa, although characterized by skin fragility and abnormal scarring, is also associated with blistering and not with hypermobile joints. The main differential diagnoses are inherited connective tissue disorders such as Ehlers–Danlos syndrome, cutis laxa, Marfan's syndrome, and pseudoxanthoma elasticum.

! Beighton score chart	
Manoeuvre	**Score**
Bend at the waist and place hands flat on the floor without bending knees	1
Score 1 point for each knee that will bend backwards	2
Score 1 point for each elbow that will bend backwards	2
Score 1 point for each thumb that will bend backwards to touch the forearm	2
Score 1 point for each hand if the little finger can bend backwards beyond 90º	2
Maximum score	9

The Beighton criteria are used in the assessment of hypermobile joints. The Beighton criteria combine phenotype, clinical history and symptoms as well as the above score. A high Beighton score is highly suggestive of joint hypermobility.

At least six different phenotypes of Ehlers–Danlos syndrome are classified; however, there is a great deal of overlap between them and absolute clinical distinction is difficult. The complications of Ehlers–Danlos syndrome are varied and include vascular complications (fortunately rare). The vascular form may be complicated by catastrophic arterial rupture and phenotypically shares some marfanoid (facies and habitus) and osteogenesis imperfecta (osteoporosis) features. The history (including premature delivery) for this child is most suggestive of classical (type I or II) Ehlers–Danlos disease.

The presence of cardiovascular disease (e.g. mitral valve disease and/or aneurysms) and dental disease should be formally assessed. Most forms of Ehlers–Danlos syndrome are associated with a normal life-expectancy, although lifestyle may be restricted. Hypermobility can be the major cause of disability and requires support, physical and occupational therapy as well as appropriate pain management. Other family members should be assessed for features of this autosomal dominant syndrome complex.

KEY POINTS

- Ehlers–Danlos syndrome is characterized by varying degrees of skin laxity and fragility, with easy bruising and abnormal atrophic scars, as well as joint hypermobility.
- It is frequently unrecognized and the diagnosis may only come to light after non-accidental injury has been considered.
- The cutaneous features may be disfiguring, however the joint disease can be disabling.

INDEX

References are by case number with relevant page number(s) following in brackets. References with a page range e.g. 25(68–70) indicate that although the subject may be mentioned only on one page, it concerns the whole case.